Caring and Well-being

Something is missing in contemporary health and social care. Health and illness is often measured in policy documents in economic terms, and clinical outcomes are enmeshed in statistical data, with the patient's experience left to one side. This stimulating book is concerned with how to humanise health and social care and keep the person at the centre of practice.

Caring and Well-Being opens by articulating Galvin and Todres' innovative framework for humanising health care and closes with a synthesis of their argument and a discussion of how this can be applied in health care policy and practice. It:

- presents an innovative lifeworld-led approach to the humanisation of care;
- explores the concept of well-being and its relationship to suffering and outlines the rationale for a focus on them within this approach;
- discusses how the framework can be applied and how health and social practitioners can draw on aesthetic and empathic avenues to help develop their capacity for care;
- provides direction for policy, practice and education.

Investigating what it means to be human in a health and social care context and what the things that make us feel more human are, this book presents new perspectives about how professionals can enhance their capacity for humanly sensitive care. It is a valuable work for all those interested in ideas about care and caring in a health and social context, including psychologists, doctors and nurses.

Kathleen Galvin is Professor of Nursing Practice in the Faculty of Health and Social Care, University of Hull, UK.

Les Todres is a clinical psychologist and Professor of Health Philosophy at the School of Health and Social Care, Bournemouth University, UK.

'I congratulate Galvin and Todres for placing well-being and the person, with all of his or her complexities, at the center of our discipline. Caring and *Well-being: A Lifeworld Approach* is a milestone that will significantly shake nursing, moving our profession firmly into the domain of humanized health care. It is a must-read for every nurse academic, student and clinician.' – *Janice M. Morse, Professor and Barnes Presidential Endowed Chair at the University of Utah College of Nursing, USA; Professor Emeritus, University of Alberta, Canada; and Honorary Professor, Bournemouth University, UK.*

'This book is philosophically grounded, clinically relevant, informed by the best of qualitative research, and written with a genuine concern for the well-being of patients as well as the professionals who provide care for them. Galvin and Todres demonstrate how a solid understanding of patients as persons is both humane and eminently practical. "Caring and Well-being" is far more than a critique of how the relational and social aspects of care are overshadowed by the technical. It is a powerful guide for how we can move forward and create a healthier approach to treatment. The authors are practitioners and researchers who care deeply, have studied these issues thoroughly, and who in clear and eloquent prose remind us of what is at the heart of working in a caring and thoughtful way with patients.' – *Steen Halling, Professor of Psychology, Seattle University, USA.*

'Galvin and Todres offer a bold and passionately humane approach to healthcare. Their call to counterbalance the efficiency-driven, technology-based culture of healthcare with an emphasis on the experience of illness and suffering is timely and well-placed. Their approach is philosophically sophisticated, rooted in real-life healthcare practice, and genuinely innovative. In particular, their emphasis on seeing health as part of wellbeing and illness as part of the broader notion of suffering, demonstrates the philosophical innovation of their work. Their proposal to develop a 'lifeworld-led health-care' (contrasted with 'patient-led care') and to understand illness in terms of existential homelessness turns attention to the pressing need to offer healthcare that is not just patient-centred, but one that is also engaged with the existential dimensions of illness and is authentically compassionate.' – *Havi Carel, Senior Lecturer in Philosophy, UWE, Bristol, Author of Illness and Life and Death in Freud and Heidegger and co-editor of Health, Illness and Disease.*

'This book is a significant and scholarly contribution to the health sciences, founded on a theoretical treatise developed over several years by Galvin and Todres. The text presents a conceptual framework that articulates alternative ways to approach health-related caring and well-being in order to create a basis for more humanised forms of health-care delivery. The work derides the reductionist view of the body as dehumanising and instead offers an

alternative view via a value-base that "does justice" to the breadth and depth of being human.

The work draws extensively on epistemological and ontological tenets that are central to phenomenological and existential philosophy, as well as offering significant contributions from qualitative health and social science research, including that of the authors.

In doing so, Galvin and Todres provide an eloquent model of life-world led care, one that involves conceptualising eight humanising dimensions that are meaningfully contrasted against those considered dehumanising. It is a lively and thought provoking exploration of what constitutes our notion of well-being and offers a critical analysis of our capacity to care.

This book is designed to promote sensitivity to the human complexities of care among health professionals by providing a "helpful coherent value base for guiding practice". It does this in light of the more personalised dimensions of care that appear to be becoming less obvious in favour of economic imperatives. With this in mind, the book is acutely timely. It presents a world view that those of us who are phenomenological converts have known for a long time as one that is particularly relevant to caring practices.

There is no doubt this book has readability and resonance. Based on some highly theoretical concepts Galvin and Todres make compelling arguments for an approach to care that is easily accessible and applicable.' – *Professor Sally Borbasi, Associate Dean Learning and Teaching, Faculty of Health Sciences, Australian Catholic University, Australia.*

'In *Caring and Well-being: A Lifeworld Approach* Kathleen Galvin and Les Todres present a creative, complex, and coherent investigation of philo-sophical and practice-based perspectives on caring for others in humane, holistic, and hopeful ways. With an emphasis on innovation, contemplation, and imagination, Galvin and Todres elucidate how experience, embodiment, empathy, emotions, and ethics are all inextricably connected to promoting caring and well-being in ways that honour the lived and living experiences of human beings who cannot be reduced to charts and statistics. In the spirit of contemporary hermeneutic inquiry, this book is nuanced and evocative, insightful and inspiring, philosophical and poetic. By carefully investigating the intersections between ethics and aesthetics, policy and practice, knowledge and discourse, empathy and action, Galvin and Todres have composed a remarkable book that exemplifies their commitment to nurturing integrated lifeworld approaches to well-being in the caring professions and disciplines.' – *Carl Leggo, poet and professor, University of British Columbia, Vancouver, Canada.*

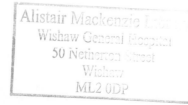

Routledge Studies in the Sociology of Health and Illness

Available titles include:

Dimensions of Pain
Humanities and Social Science Perspectives
Edited by Lisa Folkmarson Käll

Caring and Well-being
A Lifeworld Approach
Kathleen Galvin and Les Todres

Aging Men, Masculinities and Modern Medicine
Edited by Antje Kampf, Barbara L. Marshall and Alan Petersen

Forthcoming titles:

Domestic Violence in Diverse Contexts
A Re-examination of Gender
Sarah Wendt and Lana Zannettino

Turning Troubles into Problems
Policy and Practice in Human Services
Edited by Jaber F. Gubrium and Margaretha Jarvinen

Caring and Well-being
A Lifeworld Approach

Kathleen Galvin and Les Todres

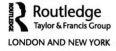

Routledge
Taylor & Francis Group

LONDON AND NEW YORK

First published 2013
by Routledge
2 Park Square, Milton Park, Abingdon, Oxon, OX14 4RN

Simultaneously published in the USA and Canada
by Routledge
711 Third Avenue, New York, NY 10017

Routledge is an imprint of the Taylor & Francis Group, an informa business

British Library Cataloguing in Publication Data
A catalogue record for this book is available from the British Library

Library of Congress Cataloging-in-Publication Data
Galvin, Kathleen M.
Caring and well-being: a lifeworld approach / Kathleen Galvin and Les Todres.
    p. cm. – (Routledge studies in the sociology of health and illness)
    1. Public health–Social aspects. 2. Social medicine. 3. Health–Social
aspects. I. Todres, Les, 1953– II. Title.
    RA418.G36 2013
    362.1–dc23   2012017737

ISBN13: 978–0–415–50460–7 (hbk)
ISBN13: 978–0–203–08289–8 (ebk)

Typeset in Sabon by
Swales & Willis Ltd, Exeter, Devon

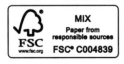

To Bill, Olivia and Sorcha – always
'my buoyancy and my holding' – Kate

To Louise, Mathew and Damian –
deep roots, expansive branches – Les

Contents

List of illustrations   xi
Preface and acknowledgements   xiii

Introduction: The need for humanised care   1

PART I
Humanising health care: A lifeworld approach   5

1 A value framework for the humanisation of care   9

2 A lifeworld approach: Revisiting a humanising philosophy
   that provides an experiential context for considering
   health and illness   23

3 Lifeworld-led health care is more than patient-led care   36

4 Caring for a partner with Alzheimer's: An illustration of
   research-based knowledge for lifeworld-led care   46

PART II
Well-being and suffering: The focus of care   65

5 An existential theory of well-being: 'Dwelling-mobility'   69

6 Kinds of well-being: Eighteen directions for caring   78

7 Kinds of suffering: Caring for vulnerability   98

8 An illustration of well-being as dwelling-mobility:
   Older peoples' experiences of living in rural areas   116

PART III
Developing the capacity to care   **131**

 9 The creativity of 'unspecialisation': Contemplative
    knowledge and practical wisdom   135

10 Complex knowledge to underpin caring: Embodied
    relational understanding   147

11 Embodied interpretation: One way of re-presenting
    research findings that may serve to sensitise the
    empathic imagination   158

12 Embodying nursing open-heartedness: An illustration
    of a core capacity for caring   170

13 Conclusion: Caring for well-being   182

    References   184
    Index   197

Illustrations

Figures

1.1 The reciprocal relationship between a humanising framework for
    care and qualitative research.   21
2.1 The boundaries and parameters of lifeworld-led care.   33

Tables

1.1 Conceptual framework of the dimensions of humanisation   11
6.1 'Dwelling-mobility' lattice   80
7.1 A framework for delineating different kinds and levels of suffering 99
8.1 Example interview questions   119
8.2 Meaning unit transformed to essential language (transformed
    meaning unit)   120

Preface and acknowledgements

We are a nurse and a psychologist who, over the last ten years, have been motivated by a coherent theme: the concern to humanise health and social care. Over this period we have published several papers in academic journals regarding this common theme that we now wish to articulate further in this book. Here we re-present these articles with some new material within the context of a thematic unifying narrative. We begin by articulating an innovative approach to 'humanising' health and social care that includes a) a conceptual framework for the humanisation of care centrally informed by 'the lifeworld' as articulated in the continental philosophical tradition b) a consideration of the importance of a focus on human well-being and suffering, c) some indications about how these concerns can inform practice by drawing on more aesthetic and empathic avenues for practitioners to engage with. Within this spirit, there are three sections to this book:

Part I – Humanising health care: A lifeworld approach.
Part II – Well-being and suffering: The focus of care.
Part III – Developing the capacity to care.

Along the way we touch upon some topical questions, for example: What do we mean by well-being? Why is lifeworld-led care more than patient-led care? How can professionals' capacity for care benefit from an engagement with the arts and humanities?

We conclude by offering a distinctive conceptual framework that integrates the humanisation of care (value and strategy), well-being and suffering (focus of care), and capacity for care (personal professional understandings) from a lifeworld perspective. These projects may all be integrated within the central notion: caring for well-being.

We are grateful to the pioneers of the phenomenological movement for inspiration and ongoing metaphorical conversations: to Husserl, Heidegger, Merleau-Ponty, Gadamer and Levinas. We are particularly indebted to the philosophical contributions of Eugene Gendlin, whose meditations on 'entry into the implicit' and embodied knowing has been pivotal for the development of our own style of 'experiential phenomenology'.

We would like to particularly express our gratitude to our companions in phenomenology who have encouraged, influenced, and supported us over the years, both through the International Human Science Research Community and through our collaborations in Sweden and the UK: Karin Dahlberg, Margaretha Ekeberg, Lise-Lotte Ozolins; Ulrica Horberg, Steen Halling, Amedeo Giorgi, Scott Churchill, Virginia Eatough, Linda Finlay, Don Polkinghorne, Kevin Krycka, Peter Ashworth, Finn Hansen, Robert Mugerauer, Robert Romanyshyn, Peter Willis, Sally Borbasi, Bernd Jager, Bep Mook, Russell Walsh, Rosemarie Anderson, Dermot Moran, Havi Carel, Tone Saevi, Carina Henriksson, Norm Friedman, Carl Leggo, Monica Prendergast and Frances Rapport. We would like to thank our colleagues and friends at Bournemouth University for coffee and discussions: Immy Holloway, Kip Jones, Fran Biley, Caroline Ellis-Hill, Karen Rees, Steve Keen, Marilyn Cash, Lorraine Brown, Sean Beer, Ann Hemingway, Steve Ersser, Clive Andrewes, Catherine Lamont, Stephen Wallace, Elizabeth Rosser, Maggie Hutchings, Andy Pulman, Anne Quinney, Regina Hess, Jan Mojsa, Vicky Rice Weber.

Finally we would like to express our appreciation to Grace McInnes and James Watson at Routledge for steering the book towards its completion.

Publication acknowledgements

The original sources of the material in this book are as follows:

Chapter 1 is a revised version of a journal article that originally appeared as: Todres, L., Galvin, K. & Holloway, I. (2009). The humanisation of healthcare: A value framework for Qualitative Research. *International Journal of Qualitative Studies on Health and Well-being*, 4 (2), 68–77. [An open access publication: Co-Action, formerly Taylor & Francis Group.]

Chapter 2 is a revised version of:
Todres, L., Galvin, K. & Dahlberg, K. (2006). Lifeworld-led care: Revisiting a humanizing philosophy that integrates emerging trends. *Medicine, Health Care and Philosophy*, 10 (1), 53–63. [Reprinted by permission of Springer Publications.]

Chapter 3 is a revised version of:
Dahlberg, K., Todres, L. & Galvin, K. (2009). Lifeworld-led healthcare is more than patient-led care: The need for an existential theory of well-being. *Medicine, Healthcare and Philosophy*, 12, 265–271. [Reprinted by permission of Springer Publications.]

Chapter 4 is a revised version of:
Todres, L. & Galvin, K. (2006). Caring for a partner with Alzheimer's: Intimacy, loss and the life that is possible. *QHW: International Journal of*

Qualitative Studies on Health and Well-Being, 1, 50–56. [An open access publication: Co-Action, formerly Taylor & Francis Group.]

Chapter 5 is a revised version of:
Todres, L. & Galvin, K.T. (2010). "Dwelling-mobility": An existential theory of well-being. *International Journal of Qualitative Studies on Health and Well-being,* 5, 5444. doi: 10.3402/qhw.v5i3.5444. [An open access publication: Co-Action.]

Chapter 6 is a revised version of:
Galvin, K.T. & Todres, L. (2011). Kinds of well-being: A conceptual framework that provides direction for caring. *International Journal of Qualitative Studies on Health and Well-being,* 6, 10362. doi: 10.3402/qhw. v6i4.10362. [An open access publication: Co-Action.]

Chapter 7 is a new chapter written for this book.

Chapter 8 is a revised version of:
Todres, L. & Galvin, K.T. (2012). 'In the middle of everywhere': A phenomenological study of mobility and dwelling amongst rural elders. *Phenomenology and Practice,* 5 (1). [An open access publication available at http://www.phandpr.org/index.php/pandp]

Chapter 9 is a revised version of:
Galvin, K. & Todres, L. (2007). The creativity of 'unspecialisation': A contemplative direction for integrative scholarly practice. *Phenomenology and Practice,* 1 (1), 31–46. [An open access publication available at http://www.phandpr.org/index.php/pandp]

Chapter 10 is a revised version of:
Galvin, K.T. & Todres, L. (2011). Research based empathic knowledge for nursing: A translational strategy for disseminating phenomenological research findings to provide evidence for caring practice. *International Journal of Nursing Studies,* 48, 522–530. doi:10.1016/j.ijnurstu.2010.08.009. [Reprinted by permission of Elsevier Ltd.]

Chapter 11 is a revised version of:
Todres, L. & Galvin, K.T. (2008). Embodied Interpretation: A novel way of evocatively re-presenting meanings in phenomenological research. *Qualitative Research,* 8 (5), 568–583. [Reprinted with permission from Sage under their standard policies and contributor agreement.]

Chapter 12 is a revised version of:
Galvin, K.T. & Todres, L. (2009). Embodying nursing openheartedness: An existential perspective. *Journal of Holistic Nursing,* 27 (2), 141–149.

[Reprinted with permission from Sage under their standard policies and contributor agreement.]

Chapter 13 is a new chapter written for this book.

Introduction
The need for humanised care

We believe that something is missing in health and social care. For example, in August 2009, a published Patient's Association report, *Patients . . . not Numbers, People . . . not Statistics,* questioned standards of care on a human level (The Patients Association, 2009; see also Commission on Dignity in Care, 2012; Cornwell & Goodrich, 2009; Parliamentary and Health Service Ombudsman, 2011). Patients and service users are telling us in different ways that they do not feel fully met as human persons in the way that care is organised and practised. These human dimensions are very important to them, and are often felt to be sometimes obscured by a service culture that has increasingly given primacy to targets, narrow and specialised outcomes, technology, efficiency drives and audit pathways. In other words people are seen as categories and often respond with the heartfelt question: where am I in all of this? The struggle that people and practitioners are intuitively identifying concerns the challenge of how to hold onto something less measurable but keenly felt. This intelligent feeling appears to be telling them that something important is in danger of being lost when overly relying on technological solutions for covering crucial dimensions of what care means to them. It is in this context that the theme of humanisation strikes a chord when it is articulated as 'those things which make us feel more human'. Further, this theme concerning 'something missing' also appears to resonate more broadly within our contemporary culture as there seems to be a significant degree of disillusionment with practices that have prioritised narrow outcomes over more meaningful human processes and well-being issues.

It is in response to this incompletely articulated 'sense of something missing' that we felt called upon to respond to. We offer a conceptual framework by which humanisation – the notion of upholding a particular view or value of what it means to be human – can be understood in a health and social care context. In developing a conceptual framework for the humanisation of care we wish to emphasise that these dimensions are the things that make us feel more human, and that such a feeling is a crucial dimension of what needs to be attended to in any practice that seeks to merit the term 'care'. It is not that we wish to deny the great achievements of medical technology and specialisation. But we do want to argue that care is much more than cure and that a care that does not attend to these human experiential processes is incomplete and can even be experienced as a 'non-care'. Later in the book we will demonstrate how this concern to focus on the *feeling of being human* is more complex than those of the person-centred care movement (which has emphasised increased choice). We will show how this latter approach may be 'too quick' to move away from *all the complex ways* that enhance or detract from the elusive experience of 'feeling more human'. Within the context of health and social care, the complexity of such a 'human care' requires a view in which illness is continuous with the broader issue of suffering, and in which health is continuous with the broader issue of well-being. Restoring such seamless connectivity where the compartments of our lives cannot be simply separated, clarifies a potentially challenging but productive focus for humanly sensitive care, namely: caring for well-being. And as a scientific, academic, and practice community, we are only in the beginning phases of articulating our knowledge of what well-being is in a positive sense, rather than being merely the absence of illness. This is why the second part of our book will offer a new perspective on well-being and suffering.

There is an increasing acknowledgement of the need to focus on well-being and not just on ill health. Within this growing discourse there is evidence to support the notion that, increasing the well-being of individuals and groups acts as an important resource in addition to directly addressing the eradication of ill health (Cox, Fulford & Campbell, 2007; Dahlberg & Segesten, 2010; Nussbaum & Sen, 1993). There have been few attempts however to define well-being in a positive sense rather than just as the absence of illness. We offer a new perspective that articulates a number of kinds and levels of well-being and suffering that need to be attended to, and show how care could be informed by a humanisation agenda.

Our focus on the *meaning* of care, and the *meaning* of well-being and suffering has been well served by a philosophical foundation grounded in the phenomenological movement (Moran, 2000; Spiegelberg, 1981), in particular Husserl's later writings on the nature of the lifeworld and Heidegger's later writings on dwelling and existential homelessness. Husserl's meditations on the nature of the lifeworld helped us to think about the phenomenon of human caring from the central perspective of the 'world of the person' on the receiving end of care. Such lifeworld-led care opened up for us a direction and complexity of issues that we will pursue in Part I. Heidegger's meditations on 'dwelling' and existential homelessness helped us to think about the phenomena of human well-being and suffering. This led to a productive direction for us to develop an existential theory of well-being, which we address in Part II.

In all these pursuits we have also been engaged in the question of what this all means for 'what it takes' to enhance professional capacity for humanly sensitive care. In Part III, we offer a distinctive understanding about the *kind of knowledge* that acts as a foundation to professionals for the practice of care. We call this form of knowledge 'embodied relational understanding'. As such it addresses a knowledge for the 'head, hand, and heart' that includes an integration of technical knowledge, empathic understanding and practical know-how. Second, we suggest some specific ways by which professionals can engage in the kind of personal/professional development that cultivates the capacity for humanly sensitive care. Third, we indicate how the practice of caring is not just a matter of knowing. Rather, it involves a more complex *capacity* for 'keeping the heart open' in an alive and responsive way. We illustrate the possibility of this capacity with reference to the phenomenon: 'nursing open-heartedness'.

The final chapter will provide a coherent synthesis of our distinctive approach to the humanisation of care. This framework provides a conceptual integration of humanisation as a value, well-being and suffering as a focus, and embodied relational understanding as a professional capacity. Finally, we articulate the central unifying narrative of these projects as 'caring for well-being' and locate this sensibility in the 'place' where knowing meets being. And it is in relation to 'this place' where knowing meets being that we may best characterise the deepest essence of the lifeworld perspective that underpins our approach to caring and well-being. In the early chapters, we elaborate on the meaning of this lifeworld approach, but here we would just like to indicate something about the relationship between the lifeworld and any systems of thought or language, as it cautions us to not confuse the map with the territory (Korzybski, 1995; Wilber, 1995). Without entering into an exposition of the lifeworld perspective in detail at this stage, we would simply like to make the point here that the lifeworld, in its living relationships, always exceeds the systems or thoughts that come to represent it. A respect for this 'excess' calls us to qualify the status of the detailed frameworks we offer in this book. We offer these frameworks, not as a system to be applied, but rather as a 'way of seeing' (and perhaps a way of being). It is our hope that readers may thus look through some of the lenses offered *in relation to* their own lifeworld encounters and projects.

Part I
Humanising health care
A lifeworld approach

Each part of the book will begin with an overview of that part, and how the various chapters in that section fit together into a coherent narrative.

The overview of this part of the book will provide a narrative that links the four chapters together in such a way that the focus on the humanisation of health care can be established as a core value upon which the rest of the book can be based.

As such, Part I points to a missing emphasis in health and social care, and to a distinctive framework and approach that re-emphasises values that may be sorely needed in institutions and organisations that merit the term 'care'. We thus offer a value framework for the humanisation of care, and clarify why a lifeworld approach offers a distinctive perspective that is highly conducive to this agenda.

Chapter 1 will offer a conceptual framework by which humanisation – the notion of upholding a particular view or value of what it means to be human – can be understood in a health and social care context. Eight philosophically informed dimensions for the humanisation of care are delineated, and the humanising and dehumanising elements in caring systems and interactions are considered. These humanising dimensions include insiderness, agency, uniqueness, togetherness, sense-making, sense of personal journey, sense of place and embodiment. Eight corresponding dimensions of dehumanisation are also named. These include objectification, passivity, homogenisation, isolation, loss of meaning, loss of personal journey, sense of dislocation and a reductionist view of the body. The chapter concludes by indicating the importance of underpinning health and social care with philosophies and practices that enable people to feel met as human beings, thus providing a living foundation for human dignity.

Chapter 2 introduces an important modification of person-centred care that we believe is central to the humanisation of health care. In order to do this, we revisit the potential of Husserl's notion of the lifeworld and how care led from this perspective could provide important ideas and values that are central to the humanisation of health care practice. Following Husserl, we call this approach 'lifeworld-led care' and outline how it provides ways of describing peoples' everyday lives as a context for humanising practices. In this chapter we describe the value and philosophy of lifeworld-led care for the purpose of providing a philosophically coherent foundation for caring practices. We show how lifeworld-led care is a humanising force that moderates technological progress. We begin by considering how the notion of the lifeworld can provide a much needed experiential emphasis for the ways we connect health and illness, well-being and suffering to our everyday lives. We consider a framework for lifeworld-led care that includes its core value, core perspectives, relevant indicative methodologies and main benefits. The framework is offered as a potentially broad-based approach for integrating many existing practices and trends and in the spirit of Husserl's interest in both commonality and variation, we highlight the central, less contestable foundations of lifeworld-led care, without constraining the possible varieties of confluent practices.

In Chapter 3 we elaborate further on the nature of lifeworld-led care because it is similar to, but different from, what has been called patient-led care. We offer an appreciation and critique of patient-led care as expressed in current policy and practice. Our critique focuses on how the consumerist/ citizenship emphasis in patient-led care obscures attention from a more fundamental challenge to conceptualise a deeper epistemological and onto-logical framework from where care can be led. We thus develop an alternative to patient-led care, and argue that lifeworld-led care is *more than* patient-led care.

The conceptualisation of lifeworld-led care includes an articulation of three dimensions: a philosophy of the person, a view of well-being and not just illness, and a philosophy of care that is consistent with this. Lifeworld-led care is shown to be a framework that not only provides ways to describe the kind of life concerns from which care can be led, but can also provide a direction for care by concentrating, not just on the absence of illness, but also on well-being in a positive sense. We conclude that a theory of well-being is pivotal to lifeworld-led care in that it provides a direction for care and practice that is intrinsically and positively health focused in its broadest and most substantial sense.

Chapter 4 offers a research-based illustration of how care can be informed by insights that emerge from a lifeworld perspective, that is insights that are based on the complex experiences of lives lived in interconnected and seamless ways. By means of a phenomenological case study, we consider a very challenging health condition, namely Alzheimer's disease within the context of a couple living together. Within this complex lifeworld context care needs to be considered, not just within the life of the person suffering dementia, but just as meaningfully within the partnership in their lives together. It is from this broader 'lens' on the couples' everyday life together that we see how lay knowledge (in this case the life-partner/carer) may be just as important as professional knowledge for the humanisation of care. The lifeworld themes that were of particular importance to the carer included: living with the partner's memory loss, the experience of adjusting to more limited horizons in their life together, caring engagement with changes in self-care and everyday routine, changes in their emotional relationship, the transition to living apart, and advocacy sustained by passion and know-how. These themes help to draw attention to an appreciation of intimacy, loss and 'the life that is possible' and as such, indicate just three of the multiple and complex issues that a focus on the lifeworld may open up. We argue that by engaging with the rich descriptions offered by such lifeworld perspectives, carers and professionals could be better equipped to understand and respond to these complex issues.

1 A value framework for the humanisation of care

The original paper on which this chapter is based was written in collaboration with Immy Holloway.

Research into health and health care has achieved substantial advancement in knowledge and improvements in care, through its focus on interventions, treatment and cure. On the one hand it is evident that increasing specialisation alongside technological advances and research have improved health and well-being. On the other hand there is increasing evidence in the media, and from qualitative research in particular, that the human dimensions of care can be obscured by a sometimes necessary technological and specialised focus. Charon (2006) speaks of the "vexing failures of medicine – with its relentless positivism, its damaging reductionism, its appeal to the sciences and not to the humanities in the academy, and its wholesale refusal to take into account the human dimensions of illness and healing" (p. 193).

It is our view however that this critique could be beneficially complemented by a positive attempt to provide a conceptual framework for humanising care that can provide direction for both practice and research. It is in this context that we have developed a humanising framework influenced by the existential-phenomenological tradition, and also by sociological perspectives that have illuminated phenomena such as human agency, anomie and alienation.

Our beginning place for this framework centred on a consideration of the philosophical question of 'what it means to be human'. And more specifically and experientially we meditated on the more practical question: what makes people feel more human in situations in which they receive care? In considering these two questions we have been philosophically informed by Husserl's notion of the lifeworld (1936/1970) and his exposition of their basic dimensions such as embodiment, temporality and spatiality. Further Heidegger's contemplations about human freedom, being with others and the authentic 'ownness' of self (Heidegger, 1927/1962) as well as Merleau-Ponty's (1964) ideas about body subject and body object also helped us to develop some core dimensions that could be applied to health care.

The conceptual framework that emerged articulated eight philosophically informed dimensions of humanisation, which together, constitute a comprehensive value base for considering both the potentially humanising and dehumanising elements in caring systems and interactions. In each case, we show, with reference to a number of published studies, evidence that is already consistent with the humanising focus articulated in our conceptual framework. The research we draw on also serves to illustrate how the dimensions in the framework live in practice.

In engaging with this evidence we also note a productive mutual relationship between a humanising value framework for health care and the practice of qualitative research. Thus in this chapter, in addition to introducing the conceptual framework for humanising care practices we also will show a) that this conceptual framework may provide a dedicated focus for guiding both research as well as practice (Morse, 2007), and b) that the nature of qualitative research is able to offer distinctive support to a humanising emphasis for care.

A framework for the humanisation of care

In this section we first consider what we mean when we use the term 'humanisation'. We then offer eight dimensions that articulate the essential constituents of humanisation in relation to caring. Each dimension is heuristically expressed as a continuum stretching from the term that characterises humanisation in a positive sense, through to the term that characterises the barrier to such a possibility. Even though each of the dimensions is expressed as an assertion that has an opposite for the sake of clarity, we are not suggesting any dualism here. In other words we are not claiming that one is either 'in a humanising or dehumanising moment' in an absolute sense, but rather that these bipolar concepts are suggestive of possibilities along a spectrum that have to be considered in context, and in relation to what is appropriate in the circumstance. We would thus like to emphasise that each dimension expresses a spectrum of possibilities which constitute 'ideal' types. We are not suggesting these ideal types as absolute values but rather as touchstones for awareness when considering the complexity of lived situations. As such we do not wish to overemphasise the negative value of what we have called dehumanising practices; there may be appropriate times when these are necessary for effective care. For example, in an intensive care situation patients fully accept the necessity for professionals to focus exclusively on the technological definitions of their current bodily functioning at particular phases of their treatment (Todres, Fulbrook & Albarran, 2000).

What do we mean by the term humanisation?

To be concerned with humanisation is to uphold a particular view or value of what it means to be human, and furthermore to find ways to act on this concern. Such a concern also needs to be practically translated into the more experiential issues of what practices can make people *feel* more human. The eight dimensions that are offered here are derived from these concerns and, taken together, can form a useful standard by which to judge the humanisation of care (see Table 1.1). This judgement would include two levels: the extent

Table 1.1 Conceptual framework of the dimensions of humanisation

Forms of humanisation	Forms of dehumanisation
Insiderness	Objectification
Agency	Passivity
Uniqueness	Homogenisation
Togetherness	Isolation
Sense-making	Loss of meaning
Personal journey	Loss of personal journey
Sense of place	Dislocation
Embodiment	Reductionist body

Note: This table is just to help the reader imagine each dimension along a spectrum of possibility rather than indicating an 'either/or' category in each case.

to which care addresses all eight dimensions, and the extent to which care can be located somewhere along the continuum of each dimension's positive humanising characteristic in relation to its more negative dehumanising feature. Therefore the following dimensions are not separate but imply one another. For the sake of clarity, we highlight these nuances as important because they can be differentially emphasised or de-emphasised in particular circumstances.

Dimensions of humanisation/dehumanisation

Each of the eight dimensions of humanisation and dehumanisation expresses a spectrum of possibilities. In each case the positive humanising value is first articulated, followed by how it may be obscured by a dehumanising emphasis. Dehumanisation occurs when any one or more of the humanising dimensions are *obscured to a significant degree*. We would like to note here that the dimensions of humanisation and dehumanisation are not absolutes but rather a matter of emphasis. For instance we acknowledge that forms of assessment and other health care practices which are problem solving in a technically helpful way, are important. However it is when these technical problem strategies overshadow the humanising dimension we refer to, that there is a *potential* for dehumanisation. Each of the eight dimensions clearly overlap in some respects but each emphasises something special as captured in the name of the dimension in each case. Such distinctiveness is also indicated by the choice of example from the qualitative research literature. We searched the qualitative literature for everyday examples that would illustrate something distinctive about the specific dimension. There are numerous examples in the literature that could be used, so we 'handpicked' examples (Bates, 1989) that we thought could provide some understanding of how the dimension could be relevant to practice and situations.

Insiderness/objectification

What makes each of us intimately human is that we carry a view of living life from the inside. To be human is to live in a personal world that carries a sense of how things are for the person. Only individuals themselves can be the authorities of how this inward sense is for them. Such subjectivity is central to human beings' sense of themselves. Our sense of feeling, mood and emotion is the lens by which our worlds are coloured. This provides important human textures for valuing the qualities of things. If such a dimension is neglected then something important is missing when responding to human need.

In *objectification*, people are made into objects by focusing excessively on how they fit into a diagnostic system, part of a statistical picture or any other strategy by which they are labelled and dealt with that does not fully take account of their insiderness. There is a whole psychology of how we separate ourselves from one another through dissociation by emphasising the distance between insider and outsider. For example, when nurses or doctors break bad news to a patient, sitting at the computer, they may focus the conversation on how the individuals fit with the statistics of their condition, the diagnostic category and other categories rather than attending to the meaning that the bad news has for the person. Along our spectrum, this is an everyday example of how an objectifying interaction may happen. An extreme example of objectification is Arendt's reference to the use of 'office-speak' by Nazi executioners when dealing with human beings in concentration camps while putting aside the work of the office before a family dinner (Arendt, 1963).

Another example of everyday objectification is shown by Holloway, Sofaer and Walker (2007) who examined the experiences and needs of people who suffered from chronic low back pain. Stigmatisation by 'the system' and health professionals as well as by significant others, emerged as a key theme from the narratives of participants. To be labelled as members of a group that were not only expensive to the system but also seen as 'malingers' deeply affected the perception of self and self-esteem and the behaviour of the patients. The study demonstrated that pain management programmes need to take into account the experience of participants, so that they feel valued and accepted. The study illustrates how labelling is one form of objectification.

Agency/passivity

To be human is to experience oneself as making choices and being generally held accountable for one's actions. This constitutes a sense of agency in which we do not experience ourselves as merely passive or totally determined but have the possibility of freedom to be and act within certain limits. A sense of agency appears to be very closely linked to the human sense of dignity. When agency is taken away one's sense of personhood is diminished.

In *passivity*, there is excessive emphasis on attitudes and practices that render the person passive in relation to their condition and treatment. Traditionally the medical model has emphasised a view of the person and the body as passively subjected to internal and external forces. The increasing emphasis on the user involvement movement in health and social care is in our view a reaction to an overemphasis on passivity. Through excessive passivity one is stripped of human dignity to varying degrees and this can be dehumanising. For example people with anorexia nervosa often rebel against the lack of dignity when an over concern with nutrition and weight gain infantilises them in such a way, that they are excessively watched and a sense of personal dignity becomes difficult to sustain.

What follows is an example of a study where practices have rendered individuals passive in relation to their condition and treatment. Johansson and Ekebergh (2006) described how women, who were recovering from myocardial infarct, experienced well-being through being facilitated to influence and take responsibility for their own bodies after a period of acute care that was characterised by insecurity and feeling 'pushed out' by their care situation. They are passively dependent on health care professionals and their knowledge, but need to regain control of their own health. A humanising care is actively facilitating participation in their health process. The study illustrates how everyday care can be humanised by enhancing agency through increased patient participation.

Uniqueness/homogenisation

To be human is to actualise a self that is unique; such uniqueness can never be reduced to a list of general attributes and characteristics . We are always more than the sum of the parts. No matter how much we are part of larger influences and contexts, there is something unique in space and time about this particular person in this particular moment that characterises their particular individuality.

In *homogenisation* there is excessive focus on how the uniqueness of the person is de-emphasised in favour of how they fit into a particular group. In their concern to please, patients agree to looking at themselves or accepting practices in which their own uniqueness is de-emphasised, and so there is a kind of self-fulfilling prophecy. When this happens, uniqueness is no longer considered by self or other.

In order to 'fit in', one may adopt the role of a 'good patient' acting according to expectations, complying with treatment and not complaining. For example there is long standing evidence that 'unpopular' patients are labelled and placed into categories and experience worse treatment (Stockwell, 1984). There is also seminal evidence of the tyranny of institutional authority: individuals develop a sick role (Parsons, 1951) and become accepting and submit to the authority of expert knowledge. This role reduces the creativity and imagination of the options that may be open to the sick person. In an early study, Rosenhan (1973) for instance, wished to show the extent of de-personalisation and labelling in institutions. His study illustrated how 'pseudo-patients actions', while under cover in psychiatric hospitals, were interpreted as pathological behaviour because of context; the 'fake' patients were not recognised.

The following qualitative study is an example of loss of unique identity and everyday practices which emphasise how individuals fit into a particular diagnosis or homogeneous group. Phenomenographic research by Widäng, Fridlund and Mårtensson (2008) showed that patients feared that they were seen as 'the disease', 'helpless', and 'an individual suffering from cancer' rather than a person with other identities, such as for instance, a 'professional woman'. The study illustrated that 'maintaining the self' and retaining personal identity as a unique individual is necessary for people during illness. In interaction with their carers, the participants found it important to keep their dignity by means of retaining 'the self' as a unique individual. This implied having some control over the situation related to what they themselves saw as important. This study illustrates the importance of a sense of personal uniqueness for well-being.

Togetherness/isolation

To be human is to be in community: our uniqueness exists in relation to others, and there is always an ongoing dialogue or 'play' between what we have in common, and how we organise and make sense of this in very personal and unique ways. Togetherness and uniqueness imply one another and make meaningful the central human experiences of both aloneness and intimacy. In different ways and in different times, privacy, human connectedness and intimacy can be important. This dimension of togetherness makes possible the experience of empathy in which we can appreciate the suffering and struggles of 'the other' who is also actively engaged in a personal world like ourselves with its own vicissitudes. Either commonality or uniqueness can be overemphasised and this has implications for care.

In *isolation* we feel ourselves separated from our sense of belonging with others. Our everyday social connections are disrupted and we can feel lonely. What we have in common with others recedes from view and we can feel like strangers. In isolation we feel alienation from others to varying degrees. It is inevitable that illness brings a sense of separation from taken-for-granted feelings of belonging with our intimate social world and significant others. Isolation however can then either be *mitigated* or *exacerbated* by different health care systems and practices. For example, any institutional bias with its sometimes necessary rules, safety procedures and concern for the efficient running of the system can take away a sense of belonging. In such circumstances a person can feel dehumanised and cut off by the creation of an alternative culture that is alien to a sense of everyday belonging. There are many practices whereby the social needs of communities with particular conditions are attended to, for example, social networking websites, special support groups. Further examples include any ways in which a person can be treated within their everyday social networks or by finding other individualised ways that can mitigate the implications of social isolation for patients.

What follows is an example of a study where practices emphasise an institutional culture that separates persons from their sense of familiar belonging. Williams and Irurita (2004), following a grounded theory study, describe a range of practices that led to isolation; participants identified feeling devalued by activities such as lack of eye contact, standing at the end of the patients' bed rather than beside them, serious or blank expressions, lack of touch, not having social conversation with the person, not remembering their personal details. In a further example, Del Barrio, Lacunza, Armendariz, Margell and Asiain (2004) have described how nurses can optimise positive experiences for liver transplant patients in intensive care by facilitating the presence of family members in the ICU at their bedside, as this qualitative study showed that the only social support that patients wanted and needed was from their immediate family. These qualitative studies illustrate how a sense of human belonging can become vulnerable in institutional contexts and the need to support such belonging in practical ways.

Sense: Making/loss of meaning

To be human is to care for the meaning of things, events and experiences for personal life. Such sense-making involves an impetus or motivation to bring things together, to find significance and to make wholes out of parts. Within this context we are story makers and storytellers. The search for narrative truth is often experienced as more humanly significant or felt to be more meaningful than the search for statistical truth. Sense-making looks for *Gestalt* and patterns that connect. When such sense-making is taken away from us in varying degrees, we can experience a sense of dislocation and meaninglessness. This can feel like being part of a machine or a 'cog in the wheel'. In finding patterns that connect for our lives we are acknowledging a certain seamlessness to living in which life cannot be essentially compartmentalised into the private and the public, concerns of body and concerns of mind, health care from social care, from economic care: human needs are holistic and transcend such differentiated discreet categories.

In *loss of meaning*, human beings can become merely numbers and statistics. When we are counted as a statistic our treatment often doesn't make sense to us, because what is important statistically does not necessarily connect with individual human experience. For example within the UK, 'a postcode lottery' has developed in which political and geographical considerations determine differential treatments. Apart from the general issue about lack of equity, in the present context, we wish to draw out the theme of 'not making sense' from the patients' perspective. It does not make sense to people with cancer living in one part of the country that they cannot get treatment the same treatment as another person living in a different part of the country.

Statistical realities can produce inequalities because they are usually based on a utilitarian philosophy and are designed for large scale representation and standardisation. When human beings are forced to fit into the standardised framework they often feel that it makes logical sense, but do not always experience practices of standardisation as systems of *care*. Within this context there is also insufficient appreciation of how different systems of care, and the agencies within them, contribute to the fragmentation of 'sense making' by the agencies and practitioners themselves feeling disconnected.

Charmaz (2006) used a grounded theory approach to examine ordinary everyday pursuits of people with chronic illness. The purpose of this was to explore how people use past and present involvement in activity to form implicit and explicit meanings of their health, well-being and emerging selves. The study described how a sample of people with chronic illnesses such as diabetes, multiple sclerosis and heart and circulatory disease measured their everyday pursuits and involvements as indicators of their health and adopted these measures as markers of who they are and who they are becoming. The research illuminates how people were able to make sense of their health and well-being by taking their focus beyond their symptoms to looking at how they are doing within their larger lifeworld contexts.

Personal journey/loss of personal journey

To be human is to be on a journey. We live forward from the past; how we are in any moment needs to be understood in the context of 'a before' and 'a next'. We move through time meaningfully and do not exist in a vacuum; to be human is to be connected to a sense of continuity. In addition, the future faces us as an unknown that offers the possibility of novelty and something different. To be human is to be connected to the familiarity of the past as well as to move into the unfamiliarity of the future. One can be oppressed by the past repeating itself and stultified by the familiarity of merely 'more of the same'. On the other hand individuals can be dislocated and shocked by the unfamiliarity of events that excessively wrench them away from the familiar. This engagement with temporality thus needs to be understood when considering a more humanised form of care; how the meaningfulness of a person's personal journey can either be supported or lost.

Loss of personal journey can happen when health care practices do not pay sufficient attention to the history and future possibility of a person's life. This manifests in an excessive emphasis on *how* the person is, not *who* the person is. For example in 'snap shot' consultations individuals are separated from their normal social context and treated as cases rather than persons with a history and biography. In health care delivery systems there is sometimes little room for considerations of continuity, or of how a person's sense of continuity is maintained. The focus is very much on the present. The trajectory of technological advances as well as demands on practitioners' time mean that a snap shot approach to health care conditions needs to be complemented, with a more biographical approach, which appreciates a person's history and importance of continuity: an increased emphasis on *who* the person is. The feeling of knowing 'who they are', helps people know and feel how their care is linked to their history. A dehumanising practice occurs also where individuals are oppressed by sameness, routine and repetitious activity. A practitioner will keep on interacting with the patient in the same way and this reduces possibilities by experiencing oneself as being 'more of the same'. Medved and Brockmier (2008) interviewed adults who had suffered brain injury to explore how people experience themselves and their sense of self following significant neurotrauma and disability. The researchers discovered that during the course of the narrative interviews with their participants, the autobiographical accounts asserted a sense of sameness and continuity for the participants even when they suffered memory impairment. The stories told evoked a sense of continuous self and an unbroken connection between pre injury and post injury self. This study underlines how people are able to attend to the tasks of achieving a sense of personal continuity even in the face of profound changes in everyday life for disabled patients.

Sense of place/dislocation

To be human is to come from a particular place; such a habitat is not just a physical environment measured in quantitative terms but a place where the feeling of at-homeness becomes meaningful. Such a sense of place is not just a collection of colours, textures and objects but rather gathers around that which constitutes the kind of belonging that provides a degree of security, comfort, familiarity, continuity and unreflective ease. When wrenched away from such a sense of place and locality, one can feel dislocated and can be made a stranger.

In *dislocation*, a form of dehumanisation occurs where a sense of place is lost or obscured and a sense of strangeness arises. In this circumstance people are challenged to find a sense of place in a new and unknown culture where norms and routines are alien to them, and where spatial re-orientation must take place if they are to fit in, similar to 'the stranger' who has a sense of dislocation when first experiencing a new place as described in the essay by Schütz (1944).

Insufficient attention is paid to the quality of space in our health care environments. Attention is needed for an architecture of space that can be conducive to privacy, dignity, homeliness and hopefulness. Furthermore spaces are not just created by physical environment alone but also by what happens within them and the practices that occur there that make the space hospitable to the richness of human life. The overspecialisation of space needs to be tempered by an attentiveness to how to bring forms of life that are fully human to the space. A study by Reed-Danahay (2001) shows how location can be important for a sense of well-being. She carried out an ethnographic study in a residential unit for people with Alzheimer's in the

United States using the concepts of place and non-place from Augé and Bourdieu. Analysis showed that some residents experienced greater confusion partly due to the bureaucratic 'office-like' and 'unhomely' setting in which they lived. In other words their confusion could not just simply be explained by the neurophysiology of Alzheimer's disease on its own, as if it occurred without a living context. Reed-Danahay thus argues that the biomedical model of Alzheimer patients pathologises their behaviour and underestimates the human dimensions of living in qualitatively different environments.

In contrast the following study considers the positive impact that an environment can have, both in terms of its architecture and the practices and routines that take place there. Arman, Rannheim, Rehnsfeldt and Wode (2008) used a phenomenological approach to explore the perspectives of sixteen patients who had experienced anthroposophic care at a specialist facility in Sweden. The patients felt that they had encountered an environment that was like a 'retreat'. The absence of visible computers, telephones and radio created a 'peaceful oasis' that was homely. This study illuminates how well-being cannot be considered separate from the atmosphere and ' rhythms' created by the built environment and the ways in which these spaces 'speaks'. This anthroposophic hospital referred to in Sweden is a distinctive example of how a more humanised form of care is supported at many levels including the architectural level. These studies underline how a 'sense of place' is crucial for a more humanising emphasis when considering health care practices.

Embodiment/reductionist view of the body

To be human means to live within the fragile limits of human embodiment. Our insiderness reveals the human body as tiredness, pain, hunger, loss of function, excitement, vitality and other experiences of the human body's being-in-the-world. When un-preoccupied with the vicissitudes of bodily attention, embodiment supports us in moving out into the world, attentive to people, places and tasks in life. On the other hand one's attention can be dominated by bodily messages that announce 'dis-ease' and are a reminder of the limits of our everyday possibilities and potentials. Consistent with this dimension, a humanising perspective will view well-being as a positive quality that makes life worthwhile and not just as an absence of illness, with the body viewed as merely an object to fix. A model of causality that is deterministic and linear can be dehumanising in that it underestimates human spirit, purpose and meaning.

In *a reductionist view of the body*, there is an overemphasis upon signs and symptoms and the body as separate from its broader contexts, and sometimes this is necessary. But in excessive reductionism there is an overemphasis on tissue, organ, hormones, electrolytes and a neglect of a more relational view of the body in its broader meaningful context such as within psychological, environmental, social, and spiritual matrices. A reductionist causality regarding the body can be dehumanising in that it can neglect the implications of 'being a person in there'. A view of biomedical causality that stresses a microanalysis of internal structures can be an overly narrow perspective when describing the complexity of meaningful relationships of living in which the body participates; this oversimplification can reduce one's more complex sense of embodiment. Conversely, when a person's embodiment is considered within its broadest meaningful relationships, their options for healing resources may be broader, and they may feel more in accord with the complexities of living. The emerging field of 'mind-body medicine', although expressed in an excessively dualistic way, is an acknowledgement of the need to consider broader causal contexts in a more comprehensive view of illness and well-being. Likewise, the increasing attention to environmental and complementary medicine similarly expresses an awareness of a broader and alternative framework of intelligibility for wellness. An example of a dehumanising interaction that is informed by a reductionist view of the body is when a professional disbelieves a patient's symptoms because the evidence for their back pain does not 'show up' in physical tests.

An empirical study from Canada demonstrates one of the ways in which less reductionistic views of the body can become important in supporting more humanising forms of care. Kontos and Naglie (2007) used performance-based presentations to help health professionals become more aware of the danger of depersonalisation when patients cannot communicate in verbal ways. Here, a view of the moving body as a realm of significant meaning becomes an important resource for humanising practices. Based on findings from focus groups with older people with Alzheimer's, they demonstrated how patients' bodily expressions could be understood in more meaningful ways. They showed how, in spite of increasing dementia, patients retained a sense of 'embodied selfhood' and how their bodies meaningfully communicated 'states of self' without words. By facilitating increased understanding of how patients communicated in bodily ways, professionals could then learn how to respond in interactive ways that confirmed the 'personhood' of the individual, even when they could no longer verbally express themselves fully. This is one example, where an understanding of non-reductionist views of the body becomes important as a humanising resource.

The reciprocal relationship between the humanising value framework and qualitative research

The eight dimensions offer a framework for distinguishing both the range of humanising issues that could be fruitfully researched, as well as an evaluative basis from which humanising and dehumanising elements can be judged along a spectrum of possibilities.

It is thus possible to imagine that a range of research programmes could include qualitative studies on all features of humanisation relevant to the eight dimensions. Therefore, for example one could imagine an interesting inter-disciplinary programme that includes architects and human geographers whereby patients' experiences are analysed in order to support the design of built facilities that are conducive to a sense of well-being and 'at-homeness'. Taking the framework as a whole with its eight dimensions also allows consideration of where research programmes may be particularly needed. For example one may find that there are many meaningful studies in the area of increasing patients' agency but a lack of studies in another important area such as 'sense-making' whereby new understandings of how patients make meaning of their illness and situations can inform professional consultations.

The framework also provides an evaluative basis from which humanising and dehumanising elements can be judged along a spectrum of possibilities. Each of the eight dimensions (such as agency/passivity) provides a particular nuance that expresses its potentially humanising and dehumanising elements in caring systems and interactions. In practice these extremes very seldom occur. However it is useful to consider the direction of movement that may be appropriate in any concrete situation. For example, in an intensive care context, Todres et al. (2000) showed that a patient became aware how, at a certain stage within the marginality of her situation, it became important for her to value the definition of her well-being in more objectified ways as given by feedback from the monitors around her. She describes a moment where she 'felt fine' but realised from the activity of the professionals that her condition was critical. At this stage she very quickly achieved a switch of perspective in which she fully valued and participated in the more objectified definitions of what was going on. At another stage however she indicated how she really needed the professionals around her to be more flexible in moving into a more humanising emphasis, which validated and nurtured a sense of her 'insiderness' and subjectivity. She became aware of how such flexibility is not often easily achieved. In providing this dimension of insiderness/objectification and research that illuminates such dilemmas, health care professionals might become more sensitive to the human complexities of care in concrete situations.

In conclusion the framework is thus able to provide a helpful coherent value base for guiding practice as well as for providing direction to a dedicated and coherent research programme.

Qualitative research: Offering distinctive support to a humanising emphasis for care

The studies used here to illustrate each of the eight humanising dimensions, give an indication of how qualitative research is particularly conducive for illuminating the complexity, depth and range of living situations relevant to more humanised forms of care. A humanising emphasis requires a particular kind of 'knowledge for care' and needs studies with certain epistemological and methodological characteristics. Such characteristics are intrinsic to qualitative research and include: a focus on the insider perspective; description, evocative impact, rich unique contextualisation rather than a premature emphasis on abstraction, and discovery orientated, open-ended enquiry.

We are thus describing a reciprocal relationship between a humanising framework for care and qualitative research that can be expressed as shown in Figure 1.1.

Conclusion

Is the humanisation of health care a luxury? We do not think so. There is increasing evidence in the media, and in our culture at large, that everyday citizens are worried that the more personal dimensions of care are being neglected in favour of 'bottom line' outcomes; the quality of the journey is just as important as the destination. So, it is not that humanisation of health care is not important; clearly it is, as evidenced by recent policy documents that highlight professional compassion, dignity in care and greater patient choice (Department of Health, 2007, 2008, 2010; Office of Department of Health, 2005; Social Care Institute for Excellence, 2008; The Patients Association, 2009). Although this policy document is within the British context, they are significant because they explicitly address the need to humanise health care. It is in this context that a dedicated focus for developing

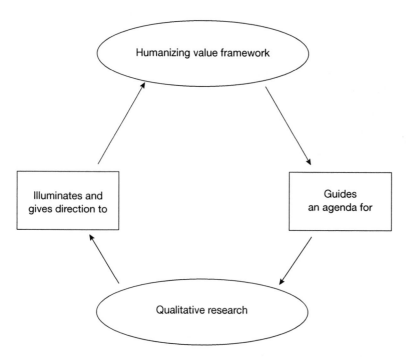

Figure 1.1 The reciprocal relationship between a humanising framework for care and qualitative research.

theoretical frameworks and research studies that support the humanisation of care may be timely. If not, existing efforts and pockets of practice that attend to humanisation may remain piecemeal as isolated practices without guidance from coherent theories and research programmes.

The philosophically informed humanising dimensions offered here may provide some positive directions by which people may feel more deeply met as dignified human beings. As such, care led from here is understood to be centrally informed from a value base that does justice to the depths and breadths of being human. And this leads us to our next chapter about a lifeworld-led care.

2 A lifeworld approach

Revisiting a humanising philosophy that provides an experiential context for considering health and illness

The original paper on which this chapter is based was written in collaboration with Karin Dahlberg.

It may be timely to review the perspective of the lifeworld as a foundation for a more humanising practice of care. This leads to the proposal of a model of lifeworld-led care that can provide a deeper philosophical context within which the more specialised approaches of biomedical conceptions of health and illness can be considered; an approach that can connect these biomedical 'views from the outside' to the more experiential 'views from the inside'. In addition we will show how a lifeworld approach can provide valuable concepts for describing health and illness situations in ways that are broader than those offered by the biomedical model, and which connect people to the more far-reaching contexts within which their everyday living takes place. This chapter may therefore serve as both an overview of this area for readers relatively new to this subject, as well as an integrating philosophical approach for a number of allied emergent practices. So, although the specific components of the arguments are not new in themselves, we believe that we offer an innovative synthesis that can inform both the value and scope of lifeworld-led care. The chapter is thus necessarily simplistic, but aims to further point the way towards this very rich tradition. (For more in-depth explorations, we would recommend Svenaeus, 2000; Toombs, 2002; Van den Berg, 1972b.)

This chapter essentially revisits the notion of the lifeworld as a possible coherent foundation for providing humanising values in the face of proliferating technology and specialisation. We do this by offering an outline of the notion of the lifeworld, and how this can provide a more holistic perspective on being human. A model of lifeworld-led care is then generated that can serve as an integrative force for a number of emerging allied practices of care.

The need to balance technologies and systems of care with humanising forces

The groundswell in movements towards user empowerment in health care (NHS Executive, 1999; Department of Health, 2002, 2005) – from user-defined health outcomes in research (Entwistle, Renfrew, Yearly, Forrester & Lamont, 1998), to patient forums and support groups, to the involvement of users in shaping services and research design (Faulkner & Thomas 2002; Trivedi & Wykes 2002), and increased participatory citizenship in general – may be seen as a response to the 'down side' of technological progress, namely its potential to foster less personal and less humanised processes, systems and institutions (Romanyshyn, 1989).

In this section we explore how the 'spirit of technology' is in need of a humanising philosophy. While this is not a new idea, it provides an important context for any argument about a philosophical foundation with humanised care as a core value.

Many writers have discussed the potentially dehumanising implications of technological progress. Heidegger (1966) was one of the early thinkers to apply himself to this topic. Essentially, he was concerned with how technological progress increased the distance between 'hand' and 'world'. By putting more elaborate 'tools' and 'processes' between the two, we face the consequences of an increasing lack of intimacy between our human experience and the world around us. Furthermore, this could affect our sense of human identity, in that we become like objects ourselves, trying to fit into impersonal systems and the production line. The up side is greater control of our environment and the objective world; the down side is a blinkered vision, concentrating our focus on 'getting there quickly' and 'getting more', quickly, whatever 'there' and 'more' are. However, human intimacy with our world requires a less means-oriented focus, where people and things are not quickly reduced to their use.

Marx (1977) took this concept of alienation further into his economic theories. He was concerned about the psychological implications of increased specialisation for our sense of human identity. He feared we were losing track of our unspecialised 'richness' and becoming more like a 'cog in the machine', a mere 'means of production'. Although his economic theories do not appear to have stood the test of time, his psychological theories about the dangers of specialisation may hold some truth in these times of becoming excessively fixed in our roles.

Habermas (1990) took both Heidegger and Marx further. In his notion of the colonisation of the lifeworld, Habermas looked at the down side of modernity, whereby capitalism and technological progress could turn humans into mere commodities, with their value determined by how efficiently they fit into larger, impersonal systems and processes, "*the tail wags the dog*".

Foucault (1973) also developed insightful analyses of how the spirit of technology could result in depersonalising and dehumanising forces, particularly in relation to medical institutions. He gave compelling arguments of how medical and technical conceptions of health and illness have become a language that is used in very powerful ways to perpetuate depersonalising and dehumanising practices of care.

As both a sociologist and cancer survivor, Frank (1995) discussed how the increasing specialisation of health care personnel, and the advancing nature of technology in medicine, obscures the attention given to caring in a more holistic way. He argues for a perspective where the fuller context of a human being's historical narrative and identity can be given proper attention.

There is also an emerging body of qualitative research studies in which patients speak of their need for more humanised approaches to their treatment. In a study about caring for a loved one with Alzheimer's disease (Galvin, Todres & Richardson, 2005), the lonely position of the carer was highlighted in the way he struggled to mediate between impersonal systems of care and his loved one's journey – this person who mattered.

In an exploration of violent encounters in psychiatric care from the perspective of the patients (Carlsson, Dahlberg, Lützen & Nyström, 2004), the researchers found that violence occurs where there is detached, impersonal caring. These encounters are experienced by the patients as uncontrolled and insecure, and therefore full of risks.

In this brief review, we have indicated the need to balance technology and systems of care with humanising forces. But what do we mean by humanising forces? To answer this, we again look to Heidegger's teacher and mentor, Edmund Husserl, who highlighted the concept of the 'lifeworld'. This notion could remind us of a coherent philosophical foundation for underpinning our perspectives and methodologies for humanising health care, and in this chapter we elaborate further on this lifeworld approach.

The lifeworld

A philosophical foundation for more humanised forms of care

Just as fish may take for granted the water they swim in, we as humans may find it difficult to notice and articulate the humanly qualitative nature of the world we live in. Ours is not a universe of neutral objects with ourselves fitting in to these physical forces; nor are we simply minds or brains that attach meaning to this neutral world of processes, others and things. Instead, there may be something more humanly intimate about the world in which we find ourselves. Husserl (1936/1970), seen as the founder of the phenomenological movement, tried to make the nature of human-world intimacy more explicit. He named this the *lifeworld*, the beginning place-flow from which we divide up our experiences into more abstract categories and names. It is a world that appears meaningfully to consciousness in its qualitative, flowing 'givenness'; not an objective world 'out there', but a humanly relational world, full of meanings. The primary nature of this relational reality means that there is no objective world in itself, nor an inner subjective world in itself; there is only a world-to-consciousness.

As well as a philosopher, Husserl was a mathematician who became increasingly concerned about how abstract, quantitative measures could forget the qualitative ground of what the numbers are about – this textured, embodied, experienced world of coloured trees, sparkling stars, alternative ways home, remembered seasons, happiness, joy, anguish and sadness. It is this lifeworld that any number (or word) refers to, without which numbers or words would have no meaning or living context (two what? three what?). Husserl was 'standing before' a pre-theoretical world-to-consciousness which is simply given to our experience pre-reflectively. He wanted to honour this pre-theoretical attitude (world-to-consciousness) and find ways to articulate what it means for who we are and our central role in bringing this world to light through the 'givenness' of experience. In this way, the lifeworld is understood as an experienced world of meaning. Any world without subjectivity, has excluded its given foundations from the beginning.

Such a qualitative world is the foundation for meaningful knowledge relevant to the humans living in and with it. Any account of events that does not start here, or does not refer to such a lifeworld description, may be forgetting its import; that is, that all events have a qualitative dimension. In health care, for example, without understanding the fullness of these qualitative dimensions, health care systems and practices may become overly concerned with partial goals and issues that measure quality in ways that are superficial and even potentially dehumanising. For now, we would like to look further at how Husserl characterised the lifeworld, and at its import.

First, the lifeworld has a holistic quality in that it is full of interrelated horizons. Any qualitative moment or event is part of a larger 'story' and 'place'; every word is said in relation to other words and meanings. Even though the interconnected horizons of meaning recede from view (or consciousness), they are implicitly there as ground from which the figure emerges (Merleau-Ponty, 1945/1962) . *Near* is in relation to *far, seen* is in relation to *hidden, self* in relation to *other*. Such relationality is primary and describes a certain intimacy in the way that qualitative life is holistically interconnected. According to Merleau-Ponty, this intimacy is different from a causal relationship, where either the world or consciousness is primary. Rather, it is best expressed as a relationship of mutual arising whereby figure and ground are often shifting and can be reversible. Any description of the significance of the lifeworld is a description of meaningful relationships within a world that is lived, thus indicating the 'more' of those relationships.

This raises a crucial question in relation to humanising health care: What relationships should be referred to when attempting to describe a world that is humanly lived? Lifeworld theory is helpful here in that it attempts to indicate the 'what' of relationships. These 'whats' refer to temporality, spatiality, intersubjectivity, embodiment and mood – dimensions that have been referred to as the constituents of the lifeworld. Husserl's consideration of these dimensions was developed further by Heidegger (1927/1962), Merleau-Ponty (1945/1962), Van den Berg (1972a) and Boss (1979). It should be noted that, in line with the holism of the lifeworld, these categories imply one another and are intertwined. However, considering each one separately has been helpful in emphasising particular nuances of lived experience. The writers cited above differed to some extent in how they named and divided up these dimensions, but all included some discussion of the following five constituents:

Temporality

Temporality refers to the continuities and discontinuities of time as it is humanly experienced. Each moment of human experience is part of a story and temporality gives human experience its 'storied' nature. The qualities of temporality are not just its quantitative, neutral 'tick-tocks', although time may sometimes be experienced like this, as we increasingly try to fit our lives into the pressures of clock time, for example. Instead, the word 'pressure' indicates only one possible variation of qualitative time. The past can come up close, and the future recede; the rhythms of the seasons can refresh or oppress. We live with time in many ways, we can have the feeling of a number of possible futures – the feeling of possibility; or we could feel the anxiety or depression of our future closing down, limiting the possibilities of living forward. Descriptions of such temporal meanings resonate with our everyday intuitions of what it is to be human. Within health care, a lifeworld description would need to include this, and not just the 'tick-tock' measures of, for example, the growth of a tumour.

Spatiality

Spatiality refers to the environing world; a world of places and things that have meaning to living. We exist in relation to what is over there in terms of spatial distance or closeness. But this distance or closeness is not primarily meaningful in its quantitative measurement, its metres and centimetres. Rather, things and situations are close or distant in terms of their significance for our daily lives. For example, when longing for a missing friend, we may ignore the pot plant that is three inches away, while the presence of the one longed-for is close in his or her absence.

This personal topography changes from moment to moment. When sick in bed and in pain, our world may shrink to the immediate environment of our room. In this mood, we may become particularly focused on the view outside the window of a dark parking space or a group of trees. When engaged in an artistic project, fallen leaves on the ground may speak of growing older. So, things in this environing world do not have simple, unequivocal meanings but have a number of potential meanings depending on where they fit into our lives at that moment. A qualitative description of human spatiality therefore includes how things appear in terms of closeness or distance, and in terms of meaning within such space. A lifeworld description that intuitively resonates with our everyday human living would include a description of how the meaning of the environing world looks or changes as circumstances change. So, for example, as we begin to feel better, the curtains no longer appear protective but start obscuring the welcome reach of daylight, inviting us outside.

Intersubjectivity

Intersubjectivity refers to how we are in a world with others. As selves, we cannot be understood without reference to how our lives take place within a social world. It is not just a people world of objects bumping into one another and reacting in mindless ways (although this can sometimes be the case). Instead, intersubjectivity means that we exist with others in an understanding way, or as Merleau-Ponty (1945/1962) puts it, we are part of an embodied world: Others are always taken into account in some way – even ignoring someone is a form of 'taking into account'. Our human capacity for language extends our intersubjectivity and social understanding in that we can share meanings and relate these meanings to our own unique situation as it unfolds. So, through intersubjectivity and language, we locate ourselves meaningfully in the ongoing interpersonal world. How we are in relation to this interpersonal world is often uppermost in our meaningful living: who I am getting on with, who I am not; worrying about Timothy, looking forward to seeing Farnaz.

When unwell, the touch of a human hand reconnects us with a sense of hope that welcomes other possibilities of interpersonal relating beyond illness, or can make us feel more remote (Van den Berg, 1955). Forms of inter-subjectivity can humanise or dehumanise us, such as kindness or violence. The nature and power of the kind of dialogue that patients and doctors engage in may thus be a central factor in healing (Svenaeus, 2000). Intersubjectivity also includes how we are in the middle of culture and tradition and how we carry this forward or differentiate ourselves from this in conscious and unconscious ways. So, a description of a person's interpersonal world may be the key to describing the relationships intrinsic to the lifeworld. We cannot fully understand the quality of an illness as it is lived, without also under-standing what it means interpersonally and culturally.

Embodiment

Embodiment refers to the concrete 'here' of ourselves. It is not just our bodies as objects to which things happen (although we do also experience our bodies like this). Embodiment refers instead to the 'lived body'; one that is not best described by chemicals and neurones but by how we bodily live in meaningful ways in relation to the world and others. The bodily self acts and positions itself in space in specific and intelligent ways – like knowing where to put our feet without thinking. Bodily, we are in a meaningful relationship with space. The bodily self feels – it does not just count its hormones, but 'melts' with love or tenses up with fear. This fluid body shapes itself emotionally to the world – the anorexic body saying 'no', not just to physical nourishment but to the dubious offers of emotional nourishment that have come to mean ownership by another.

Bodily, we are also in a primordial relationship with our interpersonal world. Others can partially constitute our bodies, for example as a commodity, and we may begin to pre-reflectively walk in a rebellious or compliant way. Body language speaks volumes. So, meanings of the lifeworld are not just thought but are embodied, going deep into the ways we expand or contract, digest, face, hold or expel the meanings of the lifeworld. Meaning is grounded in the templates of bodily existence; they give meaning to the world's textures, tastes, smells, sights and sounds. So, a description of our feeling and moving body in relation to the other three meaningful constituents should be included in any lifeworld description of intelligible living (Boss, 1979).

Intuitively, as human beings, we understand such descriptions of bodily life – they resonate well with our everyday realities. In illness, a lifeworld description would not just include a description of the 'inside' of the body as an object, i.e. its chemical interactions, but would look at how the body lives and functions meaningfully in the world. This careful description of a person's mode of meaningful embodiment can help to understand the illness in a more complete way – how it mutually interacts with its world, sometimes out-in (as in gestures of disgust about a lifeworld situation leading to digestive difficulties), and sometimes in-out (such as chronic spinal pain leading to an agoraphobic lifestyle). A description of embodied relatedness would thus extend the descriptive relationships to include their holistic meanings for spatiality, temporality and intersubjectivity.

Mood or emotional attunement

Lived experience is coloured by mood. It interpenetrates the other dimensions of the lifeworld, shaping one's spatial, temporal, intersubjective and embodied horizons. Anxiety reveals very different profiles of the world than joy or tranquillity do. In sadness, other times and spaces may be longed for – the body walking slowly. In loneliness, there is no-one there in a crowded room – little intersubjective fullness. Mood, in some way, saturates our being-in-the-world and is just as primary as spatiality, temporality, intersubjectivity and embodiment. Mood is intimate to how we find ourselves. It is a powerful messenger of the meaning of our situation: the vague feeling that something is wrong before we know it, or the feeling of how things are going in a complex interpersonal situation. Mood 'sniffs out' the situation and has already gathered the significance of things in immediate, bodily-felt ways. Mood is complex and often more than words can say. It is not just an internal happening, but is perceptual and interactive. Just as colours cannot be separated from their objects, so emotional attunement cannot be separated from the lifeworld.

More than this, emotional attunement both obscures and highlights: love prioritises our projects and values in a different way to fear. Mood thus has organising power and is a great motivator or de-motivator of directed action (and even neural, chemical and muscular pathways). So, in both illness and well-being, the description of mood as a qualitative dimension is part of a holistic, coherent understanding. Anxiety, determination, sympathy, depression and serenity, all intricately affect, and are affected by, our embodied, functional capacities. The depths, currents and waves of mood thus ask for lifeworld descriptions that include this language of tone. In this spirit, Svenaeus (2000) explicates how being ill is essentially characterised as a condition of 'unhomelikeness', alienated from the ways we can feel at home in our bodies, with others and in time and space.

Having briefly outlined the philosophical foundations of the lifeworld and how it may be relevant to a level of analysis that articulates the holistic relationships within which we are 'swimming' as human beings, we now turn to the possible significance of this for health care.

The concept of lifeworld-led care

This section explores how lifeworld-led care may be defined. The central value base of this approach may be reflected in the question: How can an understanding of the concrete, everyday experiences of people be used more centrally to underpin care?

Caring practices that are guided by this question would broaden the notion of evidence to reflect descriptions at a lifeworld level. Such understanding would be supported by a growing database of narrative and phenomeno-logical studies that express peoples' experiences of health and illness, their shared and individual journeys, and their interactions with others. Such descriptions of both breadth and depth would be guided by the constituents of lifeworld analysis as indicated above; the interaction of health and illness-related phenomena with individuals' holistic and interrelated experiences of meaning. Boss (1979) uses a lifeworld approach to demonstrate the importance and value of understanding such experiential meanings in health and illness. For example, he used a detailed case study to demonstrate how a number of symptoms of a woman with a long history of gastro-intestinal complaints could only be fully understood with reference to her life projects and concerns: her body image, her perception of her spatial and temporal horizons, and her meaningful relationships with significant others.

Understanding such lifeworld horizons goes beyond the case studies and accounts of people's experiences 'in their own words'. The tradition of phenomenological-empirical research (Churchill & Wertz, 2001) encourages a level of reflection and understanding in which both the shared and unique dimensions of peoples' experiences are communicated. It acknowledges that human experience is not just encompassed by local, private dimensions, or by common, public ones (Dahlberg, Dahlberg & Nystrom, 2008). Some of the implications of such a methodological approach are as follows:

1. That it tries to find a language that cares for the human order. This is a language that is full of human participation and that allows us as human beings to intuitively share in the phenomena described; a

language that finds the 'I in the Thou'; a language of experience on its own terms.

2. That it champions the value of the human individual as a starting point in human science. This includes a return to concrete experiences, the balance between articulating unique variations of experience with the ground that we share. The approach moves from the particular to the general, attempting to honour both levels of understanding and their complementarity (the hermeneutic circle).

3. That it remembers the freedom of the unique human occasion by expressing essences and themes, not as final and conclusive law-like absolutes, but rather as possibilities around which unique variations and actualities can occur. Truth in this perspective is thus an ongoing conversation which is not arbitrary but which is never finished and depends on questions and context.

(Todres, 2003, p. 202)

In addition to the above methodological emphasis, lifeworld-led care would also have a political emphasis: to inform care at both practice and policy levels on the basis of research-based descriptions of people's lifeworld experiences. This approach is more complex than merely obtaining users' views about services. Descriptions of experiences are more detailed and informative than an approach that relies on evaluations and judgements, whether from citizens or professionals. In health care, as a participative community, agendas may be better evaluated by the kind of transparency that is based on an empathic understanding of what people 'go through' in more descriptive terms. Further interpretations are therefore grounded in the lifeworld of actual experiences. This political dimension of lifeworld-led care would encourage the development of policies and processes to enable citizens' experiences to be more centrally incorporated into daily care arrangements.

A model of lifeworld-led care: An integrative force for emerging practices

This concluding section explores the possible scope and value of lifeworld-led care. We would not like to constrain the imagination about how the value and philosophy of lifeworld-led care could be translated into practice. A number of methodologies and approaches that have already been developed are broadly consistent with the values of lifeworld-led care. Examples include:

*   The emerging tradition of practice-based evidence that honours the experience and judgement of clinicians and professionals in their caring practices (Polkinghorne, 2004; Rolfe, 1998; Rolfe, Freshwater & Jasper, 2001). This tradition includes supervision or reflective practice groups whereby 'empathic imagination' is used to understand health and social

care users' worlds (Ekebergh, Lepp & Dalhberg, 2004; Halling, Kunz & Rowe, 1994).

- Support groups led by users of health and social care services that facilitate mutual understanding and support, which may lead to improvements in care through shared actionable projects. (Reason, 1994).
- Ways of disseminating the findings of qualitative research to make them valuable to users and to help deepen professionals' lifeworld understanding (Mienczakowski, Smith & Morgan, 2002; Ziebland, 2004).
- Integrated approaches to assessment and care that are based on lifeworld approaches (for example, Newman, 1999; Svenaeus, 2000).
- Phenomenological and narrative studies (Ellis-Hill, Payne & Ward, 2000; Jones, 2004; Todres, 2005) that deepen our insights into a variety of lifeworld phenomena such as people's experiences of palliative care, experiences following a myocardial infarction (Johansson, Ekebergh & Dahlberg, 2003), non-caring encounters in an emergency unit (Nyström, Dahlberg & Carlsson, 2003), and midwives' experiences of their encounters with birthing women (Lundgren & Dahlberg, 2002).
- Developments that have engaged users of services as 'paraprofessional' helpers or facilitators (e.g. Abdul-Quader, 1992; Hossack, 1999).
- Educational approaches that use the 'stories', dramatic presentations of users' experiences and the arts to deepen health and social care professionals' lifeworld understanding of 'otherness' (for example, Gray, 2003).

All of the above approaches are broadly consistent with a lifeworld-led project, although there are likely to be many more examples. The clarification of a philosophically coherent foundation for lifeworld-led care as offered in this chapter may help develop further innovations. The boundaries and parameters of such lifeworld-led care are provisionally summarised in Figure 2.1.

Core value: A humanising force for health and social care that moderates technological progress

This value is based on the intuition that individual lives matter and that the quality of human life cannot be quantitatively measured or defined. This intuition and understanding is given to human beings with their subjectivity and as beings that can humanly care for self and others (the potential to see oneself in others). In relation to health and social care, this intuitive understanding knows well-being or unease intimately, from 'within' and existentially as our common human vulnerability – through change, pain, isolation or comfort. Lifeworld-led care would highlight this value as a fundamental 'touchstone' when evaluating improved processes and technologies of care.

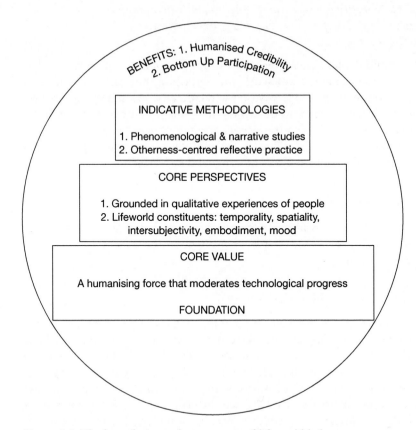

Figure 2.1 The boundaries and parameters of lifeworld-led care.

Core perspectives

Grounding: An understanding of others' worlds grounded in experiences of real people living through complex situations in holistic ways

This core perspective comes from its core value. When motivated by 'humanisation', a perspective can be opened up and pursued through intense curiosity about the descriptions of others' experiences – what things are like for them. Such openness involves a willingness to hear all the meanings and connections from others as lives that are lived. This perspective does not prematurely categorise these experiences but tries to respect their holistic interconnections as humanly meaningful stories.

Lifeworld constituents – a framework for holistic human understanding: Temporality, spatiality, intersubjectivity, embodiment, mood

The existential phenomenological tradition beginning with Husserl has provided a conceptual framework for describing human experiences in intuitively resonant ways. How we live in relation to time, space, body, others and mood is fundamental to describing the holistic context in which being human makes sense. Such a framework for human sense-making can act as a 'benchmark' for understanding health and illness; how such qualities are intimately related to the entirety of living and experiencing.

Indicative methodologies

These methodologies, while not exhaustive, are good examples of approaches that are conducive to the coherence and logic of the other components of lifeworld-led care.

Phenomenological and narrative studies

The core perspectives may be translated into a research methodology that is well suited to capturing and illuminating the experiences of self and others. Both the phenomenological and narrative research traditions pay attention to the discovery-oriented attitude of 'openness', person-centred strategies of 'data' collection, and analytical procedures and frameworks that elucidate the meaning of experiences that have been lived through in all their complexity and context (Dahlberg et al. 2008; Todres & Holloway, 2004). The findings of such studies are expressed in narrative ways to help others understand the possible shared dimensions of experiences between people, as well as their unique experiences in individual contexts.

Otherness-centred approaches for reflective practice

This kind of reflective practice may be based on cycles of reflection similar to other reflective practice approaches (see for example, Reason, 1994; Rolfe, 1998; Rolfe et al., 2001). However, within a lifeworld approach, reflecting on practice is more centrally influenced by phenomenological 'evidence' from the world of the 'cared-for', i.e. clients and patients (Beck et al., 2003), which makes this approach closer to the world of 'research' – the guidelines for phenomenological and narrative research are particularly relevant when practising an otherness-centred, lifeworld approach to reflective practice. In this approach, the emphasis is placed on the other's experience as opposed to the practitioner's or carer's self-experience. The central question in this approach is: how can practice be informed by a more in-depth understanding of the lifeworld experiences of citizens?

Benefits

The humanised credibility of relating care to real experiences

An approach that is grounded on the evidence of real experiences provides a kind of credibility that only human stories can give. Narrative truth (Spence, 1982) is different from statistical truth in that it is not merely a numerical snapshot of averages and variations but a humanly textured scene that communicates meaning and significance, and therefore carries the presence of what has happened to someone. Such textured happenings and meanings are humanising in that they are full of mood and the aesthetic qualities of living (Todres, 1998).

'Bottom-up' citizenship: Participatory democracy based on co-operative and empathic perspectives

Lifeworld-led care politically empowers citizens to own and participate in the forms of health and social care that affect them. But more than this, lifeworld emphasis can provide an 'inner life' existential view that can appeal to the 'heart' of care – the places that bind us in a common human situation, beyond economics, race and creed. This emphasis encourages co-operative strategies of working together, through a transcendence of partial 'tribal' agendas and a concern to hear the 'cries of the world'.

Conclusion

In this chapter, we began by pointing to the lifeworld as an experiential foundation for care that could complement biomedical perspectives and thus empower more humanising practices. We then outlined the theory of the lifeworld, with its roots in phenomenology. Finally, we provided an integrative framework that encompasses the core lifeworld values and perspectives, some appropriate methodologies and the relevant benefits (see Figure 2.1). As such, lifeworld-led care could offer a potentially broad-based approach for integrating many existing practices and trends that serve to humanise health care practice. The model of lifeworld-led care is offered as an orienting generalisation that highlights its core dimensions. As such it hopes to be broad enough to allow the distinct features and differences of a number of existing and emerging practices and methodologies. The methodologies suggested within the model are thus more of an indicative nature, and we can imagine much scope for variety. But in the spirit of Husserl, who was interested in both commonality and variation, we would also like to highlight the central, less contestable, foundations of lifeworld-led care: its humanising value, the holistic contextuality of lifeworld experience, and its benefits of experiential credibility and citizen empowerment.

3   Lifeworld-led health care is more than patient-led care

The original paper on which this chapter is based was written in collaboration with Karin Dahlberg.

The notion of 'Patient-centred' or 'Patient-led' care has increasingly influenced health care policy in the United Kingdom and Swedish contexts. In the midst of consumer driven concerns in both countries, the aim has been to give patients more 'choice and voice' in their own health care. Although this is a positive initiative, it has its limits and unanticipated side-effects. One implication of this trend, that may not have been sufficiently examined and understood, is how the policy documents focus implicitly or explicitly on patients as consumers (an economic emphasis) or patients as citizens (a political emphasis).

In this chapter, while appreciating the direction of patient-centred care, we offer a critique of what may be missing in both its philosophy and practice. Taking our point of departure from the previous chapter, we now develop the analysis further, and consider how the idea of lifeworld-led care can deepen an understanding of what patient-led care can mean. Our contention is that a philosophically consistent health care policy that is authentically person-centred requires attention to its conceptual foundations and would include an articulation of the following three dimensions: a philosophy of the person, a view of well-being and not just illness, and a philosophy of care that is consistent with this. We attend to these three dimensions by offering a specific view in each case:

- Philosophy of the person: an existential view of being human; *freedom and vulnerability*
- An existential view of well-being: the possibility of vitality; *peace and movement*
- Philosophy of care: how lifeworld-led care is more than patient-centred care and points to directions for practice.

An appreciation of 'patient-centred' or 'patient-led' care and a critique

In both Great Britain and Sweden, governments have realised that health care policies need to change towards more patient participation. The urge is to involve patients more in their care in general, and in particular, increase their involvement in the decisions that are to be made. We welcome this move to empower greater patient participation. This perspective that emphasises the possibility of giving more agency to people can be seen as a reaction to a historical 'medical model' approach that, in extreme forms, has over-emphasised illness and professional authority, a context that has been at risk of rendering patients as passive recipients of care. The move towards patient-centred care may thus be seen as a reaction to an image that de-emphasises patients' human agency (Hemingway, 2011).

According to *Creating a Patient-Led NHS* (Department of Health, 2005), "good practice" will involve:

- Respecting people for their knowledge and understanding of their own experience, their own clinical condition, their experience of the illness and how it impacts on their life.
- Ensuring people always feel valued by the health service and are treated with respect, dignity and compassion.
- Understanding that the best judge of their experience is the individual.
- Explaining what has happened if things go wrong and why, and agree the way forward.

These values have translated into recommendations for practice that include "better systems for 'feeding back', learning lessons", "more regular sources of information about preferences and satisfaction" and, in this context, wishes to ensure that "everything is measured by its impact on patients" (Department of Health, 2005).

What can be noticed from this approach is how such focus on systems and conditions of service give more agency to patients and ways of expressing their satisfaction or dissatisfaction. These are, no doubt, strategies that address a human need for increased agency. The question is, however, whether the meaning of health, illness, suffering and well-being is taken for granted and as such, prematurely prioritises operational and organisational concerns – an economic emphasis. In addition there may also be a prioritisation of a political view of being human that emphasises rights and empowerment. Our critique focuses on the question of what both the economic and political emphases leave out when considering the essences of health, well-being and care. We doubt that the economic and political emphasis fully encompasses the kinds of concerns and knowledge that are adequate for approaching the breadth and depth of humanly sensitive care that is relevant to us in our human health journeys. On the one hand, a consumerist/ citizenship model that overly emphasises personal or collective agency and self-authority is partial because it underemphasises patients as 'exposed' and 'vulnerable'. On the other hand, there have been reductionist versions of a medical model that overemphasises illness and underemphasises the phenomenon of human agency. When people become patients they want to be seen in *both* their agency and vulnerability and feel unmet by interactions that emphasise one or the other.

Our aim in this chapter is to present an alternative perspective that uses lifeworld theory as a philosophical framework and that can encompass both agency and vulnerability without prioritising one or the other. We believe that many practitioners already live according to some of the values and philosophical assumptions that are made explicit in this chapter. However, a more explicit articulation of lifeworld-led care as a coherent approach may provide some interesting directions for joined-up thinking and practices.

A lifeworld-led care approach

The lifeworld-led care approach that we developed in the previous chapter is here further developed by a consideration of how it is fruitfully underpinned by an existential view of being human. Like others before us (e.g. Frank, 1995; Svenaeus, 2000; Toombs, 1993), our aim is to interpret these philosophical ideas in favour of an understanding of care that acknowledges the complexities of personhood, health and illness.

In the earlier chapter, we developed a model to describe the core dimensions of lifeworld-led care. We considered how lifeworld theory and the existential dimensions of temporality, spatiality, embodiment, intersubjectivity and mood could form the parameters from which the lifeworlds of people could be understood, and further, how these descriptions could become more central in leading care. We now offer two further developments that are consistent with lifeworld-led care: An existential view of being human, and an existential view of well-being. Such a knowledge base may provide substance to an approach to care that can accommodate both human agency and human vulnerability. These developments are needed in order to indicate the *direction* of the knowledge base from which any lifeworld-led care would proceed and as such, addresses the partialities of both a consumerist view on the one hand and a narrowly biomedical view on the other.

An existential view of being human

Entering the phenomenological realm we do not fundamentally find our lives as unrelated compartments such as 'health', 'illness', 'emotional life' 'spiritual life'. Neither do we find mind-in-itself or body-in-itself. We rather find the seamlessness of everyday life and its qualitative character. In examining everyday life in its qualitative character, phenomenological philosophers such as Heidegger and Merleau-Ponty articulate a view of human being in which persons are not just other objects that are purely determined by 'natural forces'. Rather, there is an existential freedom that makes choice and agency meaningful within certain limits.

Another way of putting this is that we are beings that can transcend our determined circumstances in some sense. This reveals a view of being human that is always 'in process', and 'not finished'. This 'being in process' provides a certain openness to the ways we respond and change in response to our journeys' circumstances. On the other hand, as Heidegger (1927/1962) demonstrates, this is not to say that we are given an absolute freedom, but rather, a situated freedom. We are not separate from our concrete engagements with the world or with others, and this announces certain limitations and vulnerabilities about what we come up against: the facticity of our finitude or death, the fragilities of our bodies, the vicissitudes of existing (or living) in a particular time, place, culture and language.

Both the vulnerabilities of being human and the possible freedoms of being human are acknowledged as fundamental dimensions that are in creative tension with one another (Todres, 2007). To quote Heidegger (1927/1962, p. 435): "Once one has grasped the finitude of one's existence it snatches one back from the endless multiplicity of possibilities which offer themselves as closest to one".

Our human heritage, which means participating in this ambiguous realm in a seamless way, includes a tension between the ways that we are limited ('thrown') and ways that we are free ('creative'). Such an existential view of being human is important in that it provides a perspective by which lifeworld-sensitive care can be led. This perspective emphasises an understanding of being human in which health is conceptualised in terms of both its limitations *and* possibilities for human existence. The kind of knowledge base that is required to lead care is then more than just political or technical, but describes a philosophical understanding of how well-being and illness are intimately bound up in the human condition. Thus, we come to the need for a theory of well-being that is consistent with this philosophy.

An existential view of well-being

Without an explicit understanding of well-being, which includes the existential dimensions of freedom and vulnerability, health care policies and practice may be in danger of unreflectively assuming that health is just the absence of illness. An approach that highlights a consideration of well-being also mitigates against the trap of seeing patients as merely consumers of services. In this analysis, Heidegger's and Merleau-Ponty's reflections on the existential possibilities of being human have convinced us of the importance of including and understanding people's capacities for interpersonal intimacy and individuality of expression and creativity. Illness or pathology can thus be understood as a truncation of such existential possibilities, a closing down of our potential to exercise one's engagement with the world and the future in all the ways that may beckon (cf. Svenaeus, 2000; Toombs, 1993). An existential view of well-being refers to the possibility of well-being before it is subdivided into different domains of well-being such as social well-being, economic well-being, political well-being. Rather, it focuses on what makes well-being an experiential possibility, so that its various forms can be recognised. Such a conception of well-being as a whole may be important when promoting health and preventing illness and suffering (Nordenfelt, 1995).

Vitality, movement and peace

The existential and lifeworld-oriented view of well-being that we propose considers the inclusion of vitality, movement and peace as cornerstones, as well as the idea of meaningful life projects. These ideas arise from the previously discussed philosophical view of being human and its existential notions of freedom and vulnerability. The experience of well-being means an existence that is characterised by vitality, which encompasses the possibilities of movement and the possibilities of peace. Further, in a phenomenological understanding of vitality, movement is but the other side of peace, as peace is the other side of movement. Movement and peace should not be understood as pure opposites, since peace can be the origin of movement and movement can be the origin of peace (Dahlberg, 2008).

Movement

Well-being as vitality means the capacity for movement in a sense of being able to move into possibilities of engagement that connect us with others, other spaces, other times and other moods. We thus also refer to this form of vitality as 'existential mobility'. Heidegger (1927/1962) and Merleau-Ponty (1945/1962,1964/1968, 1960/1987) identified the existential ways in which we can move vitally into different qualitative spaces, different relationships with time, different relationships with others, different embodied movements and different moods that colour the world in different ways. Human being exists in movement, Merleau-Ponty (1960/1987) argues, and continues to say that "the world and Being hold together only in movement, it is only in this way that all things can be together" (p. 22). A view of well-being that includes the notion of a sense of vitality would thus consider all the ways in which a person is 'stuck' from, or able to actualise (or 'flow with'), these different potentials for living forward.

Smith and Lloyd (2006) pursue a phenomenology of vitality in order to describe the meaning of health. Doing that, they touch upon life as movement (Sheets-Johnstone, 1999). Within this context, health means 'to be able to'; to be able to live and carry out one's major and minor life projects. Smith and Lloyd draw on "the measures of vitality . . . from the perspective of the living, breathing, moving person who seeks wellness and a healthy and active lifestyle" (p. 263). In health and well-being we live rhythmically and in balance; we inhale and exhale, we open and close our eyes, mouths and fists, we are active and we seek stillness. Health is characterised by vital, rhythmic movement, while in illness, the movements may be broken, uneven, unbalanced, or just too slow or too quick. In focusing on the movement dimension we would like to offer two examples of well-being as vitality in movement: In the first example, one can imagine a woman with Alzheimer's disease who has lost her recent memory. When she however is taken for a walk in a much-loved garden she reconnects with much older memories, which gives her a sense of some continuity and a feeling of wellness. She finds a sense of a movement that is possible within her illness. A second example is provided by a study of dementia (Svanström, 2008): moving around the kitchen and cooking together with a young relative, set a woman with Alzheimer's on the intentional path in which she again recognised the kitchen equipment and its use, something she could not do the day before when she was by herself. Both examples show how the persons could find a sense of vitality and movement that was possible even within severe illness.

In writing about the 'Psychology of the Sick Bed', Van den Berg (1972a) describes how a bed ridden person may know the rhythm of the year more intensely than when she was up and about. A certain kind of awareness of movement is opened up to her in that the smaller movements of a growing flower and first flight of the sparrows outside the window become more significant. We thus see that movement as well-being is subtle, and more than just the physical condition of the illness.

Peace

The understanding of well-being that we offer draws further on vitality as the possibility of peace. Peace refers to a notion of stillness whether the stillness means to be restful, accepting what is present at hand, or an experience of 'letting-be'. Peace involves the full spectrum of temporality, although it is primarily present-centred. In other words, peace is essentially a coming to terms with, and even 'a welcoming' of the present moment. This does not exclude the full spectrum of temporality in that peace also involves a coming to terms with 'what has been' (past), as well as 'what might happen' (future).

From the view of vitality as peace, well-being is metaphorically illuminated as an experience of 'settling' and 'being at home', where one comes to rest with present health conditions. But more than this, it is also coming to rest more existentially with 'how things are', forgiving life its changes. For example, Johansson (2008) and Bremer, Dahlberg and Sandman (2009) describe how people who have survived cardiac arrest went on living with an existential sense of insecurity, but how they also could rearrange their everyday lives to form some peace. Sometimes they even found a better quality of life than before the illness entered. By actively confronting these threats against well-being and existence, feelings of confidence and joy of life were strengthened. Not least, the returning to everyday activities was found to give existence stability and clarity, and contributed to an important sense of coherence. A quote from one of their interviewees makes the meaning explicit:

> If we compare what I have now, then I have, then . . . now it's completely different, you could say I am living another life. Now I am living at my own pace, you know, and I am doing whatever I want during the day. I can go there if I want . . . yes, and I have more [time] with the family, the grandchildren, all of that. So, it's not even possible to compare! It's

much more fun to live nowadays than [laughter] before, so to speak. Because, at that time it was stressful and one had to work on one's back, you know.

Heidegger (1959/1966) describes 'letting-be-ness' in a way that we understand as existential sources of peace or stillness. His idea refers to the potential we have as human beings to let go of our wilfulness and to reconcile ourselves with whatever life is possible in spite of its limits. The importance of this in practical terms is that human beings who experience losses and suffer from illness can still find possibilities for well-being and a good life. Even with illness, suffering and weakened movement, there is still the possibility of peace as one source of well-being. We offer two examples of enhancing well-being through stillness.

In a number of psychotherapeutic situations (Todres, 2003), clients were able to 'settle down' into an acceptance of their vulnerabilities and the limits of their freedoms in different ways. In such circumstances a sense of peace and freedom was found, not so much in a feeling of what they could do in the future, but more in a feeling of acceptance of themselves and others as they are in the present. There was a 'sigh of relief' in realising that well-being was possible by simply making peace with 'what is'. In another example elaborated upon in a later chapter, a man who was becoming increasingly ill looking after his wife with Alzheimer's disease experienced a greater sense of peace in ' the small joys' that were possible in spite of the lack of possibilities announced by the illness. These small joys included doing things for their shared doing together rather than whether any kind of productive outcome occurred.

Well-being: Vitality as the intertwining of peace and movement

The view of well-being outlined here highlights the notion of vitality as the inclusion and intertwining of stillness and motion, peace and possibility. The rhythm and potential complementarity of peace and possibility overcomes common dualism and dichotomies, which see these dimensions as mutually exclusive categories. In well-being the intertwining of peace and movement means settling into the present moment and also an openness to what may come. This includes feelings of possibility, and such a possibility includes spatial or temporal movement in vital ways, as well as a feeling of settledness, of being at home with what presents itself to one. A well-being that is fully actualised as vitality would thus contain a strong quality of settling intimately into the present moment, as well as an energetic feeling of flow that comes with being open to the invitational call of the future.

However, one can also imagine forms of well-being in which one of these dimensions is emphasised and the other is in recession. For example one can imagine an energised feeling of vitality as movement, without peace being emphasised, when people are enthusiastically pursuing their goals. In such circumstances they receive confirmation that all their faculties and bodily powers are functioning well, allowing an un-preoccupied and vital movement into desired futures. On the other hand, one can also imagine a vital feeling of acceptance and peace, such as when a person with a number of aches and pains looks outside the window, watching children play. This may be enough to constitute a feeling of well-being in spite of tiredness, pain and sense of physical deterioration.

Lifeworld-led care: Towards applications for practice

In this section we wish to bring together our considerations of an existential view of the person, as 'freedom and vulnerability', together with our consideration of an existential view of well-being that includes vitality as 'movement and peace'. We wish to argue that lifeworld-led care requires knowledge that is developed out of the implications of an existential view of being human and an existential view of well-being. An existential view of being human, together with an existential view of well-being as articulated above, makes clear that there is always some vulnerability and some freedom in any condition. There are also possibilities for vitality, movement and peace in any condition. In caring for another from a lifeworld perspective we thus need to act in a way that represents all of these dimensions; only then will a human being feel 'met'.

This may sound over-ambitious and unrealistic, but what it demands from carers is to be open to the lifeworlds of their patients, to listen to their stories, to touch and be touched, without avoiding the ambiguities of existence. Several studies make explicit how such care supports patients' well-being despite illness (Nordgren, Asp & Fagerberg, 2007). Studies also show how lifeworld-led care characterised by openness and bodily presence makes it less likely for violent encounters to occur in psychiatric care settings (Carlsson, Dahlberg, Lützen & Nyström, 2004; Carlsson, Dahlberg, Dahlberg & Ekebergh, 2006).

Lifeworld-led care is thus more than patient-led or patient-centred care as it has been so far defined in policy documents. Although it can be seen as a form of patient-led and/ or patient-centred care, it is more deeply episte-mological in emphasis than the political aims of giving patients 'more voice'.

Within a perspective of lifeworld-led care we need knowledge that understands both the freedoms and vulnerabilities of peoples' journeys as they struggle with different health-related conditions. We also need knowledge of the possibilities for vitality, movement and peace; the deeper existential horizons and potentials that are possible.

As yet this kind of knowledge is not coherently and systematically present in the professional or public arena. However, there are some examples of such knowledge that articulate insightful descriptions of the meanings of different health conditions in terms of their existential limits and possibilities.

For example Källervald (2008) used a phenomenological approach with patients with malign lymphoma and their professional carers. These were patients who acknowledged the good care received. However, looking more closely into their lived experiences and stories, it was found that they suffered from not being existentially acknowledged. The carers confirmed that the existential demands were hard to deal with, that they met inner limitations but were also lacking knowledge of how to encounter these issues. The carers needed mentoring, supervision or other support to meet their own vulnerability so that they could emotionally cope with the full existential impact of what the patients were wishing to share. It remains a future task to draw on such examples to develop a collective and systematic body of knowledge at this level.

A lifeworld-led care perspective would encourage health care professionals to carry the kinds of knowledge and perspectives that understand the existential qualities that are both common and unique to various conditions as well as the knowledge about where existentially an individual 'can go' or 'reach for'. Such care will support peoples' own strategies to increase health and well-being. Professionals led by lifeworld knowledge do not therefore just offer technical solutions, but are able to offer 'paths' for the patient to step into in their life's journey. Such an interaction, if well informed, can lead to the patient feeling more 'deeply met' in both their vulnerabilities and possibilities. In all these ways, practice informed by lifeworld-led care would be a practice that is guided by a positive understanding of existential well-being (rather than the narrower pursuit of the absence of illness) as well as the humanising interactive style that is empowered by an existential view of being human.

Conclusion: Lifeworld-led care is more than 'patient-led' or 'patient-centred' care

The current emphasis on patient-as-consumer and the aspirations towards 'more choice' are positive in that such a framework places patients at the centre of care. In helpfully emphasising citizenship empowerment issues, policy moves like 'Creating a Patient-led NHS', however, directs attention away from the lifeworld and the deeper existential issues. It does not provide an encompassing framework within which the vicissitudes of peoples' lives, their wellness and suffering, can be meaningfully addressed.

A lifeworld-led care would provide a broader and deeper context within which political empowerment of patients is still cared for. It distinctively would enable health care professionals to attend to lifeworld-directed ways for caring (rather than a strategic overemphasis on patients' agency alone). Patients would be able to step forward, not just as 'consumers' competing for care, but as 'storied beings' who consult others with specialist expertise from time to time.

This is an existential partnership model that acknowledges differential levels of expertise and understanding between patient and professional (Svenaeus, 2000; Toombs, 1993). The patient can understand her/his journey better than any other and in that sense is an expert. Professionals need to acknowledge but not relinquish their expertise, and lead their care from an expanded view of knowledge as articulated above, and not just from 'technical' knowledge (Polkinghorne, 2004). This lifeworld knowledge is different from 'technical' knowledge in that it is always on the way, whereas technical knowledge is fixed until the next new evidence becomes available. It is more open than the bounded categories that are given with a diagnosis, and acknowledges the unique unfolding of a person's illness journey in relation to complex contexts.

The existential view of well-being is pivotal to lifeworld-led care in that it offers a direction for care and practice that is intrinsically positively health focused in its broadest and substantial sense. It is this view of well-being that may most crucially define why lifeworld-led care is more than patient-led or patient-centred care. As indicated earlier, a more explicit articulation of lifeworld-led care and its meanings of health, illness, suffering and well-being, may provide reflective resources for practitioners.

By highlighting well-being as a fundamental human potential for living, health-related issues are firmly recontextualised and embedded within their deeper existential matrix. Care led 'from there' is thus necessarily holistic, but more than this, directional. This directionality is provided by the view of well-being, which may be considered to be an idealistic or romantic notion in that it only appears to ever be achieved or touched on in moments and limited periods. Nevertheless, it could be argued that well-being is a fundamental motivation within the human heart, and that people invariably recognise what it is, and more crucially, its absence. Illness and well-being thus cannot be considered apart from one another. And together, they constitute a core foundation for our humanity.

4 Caring for a partner with Alzheimer's

An illustration of research-based knowledge for lifeworld-led care

In Chapter 2 we outlined the core values, core perspectives and indicative methodologies of lifeworld-led care. We indicated a number of allied approaches that are consistent with lifeworld-led care that have been developed. When discussing relevant indicative methodologies, we considered the kind of research knowledge that was particularly conducive to guiding lifeworld-led care. In this chapter we offer a research-based illustration of how care can be informed by lifeworld insights, that is, insights that are based on the complex experiences of lives lived in seamless ways. As readers will see, we show how a particular kind of phenomenological methodology is helpful in producing this kind of knowledge and thus spend some time on methodological issues before illustrating the lifeworld insights that have relevance to practice. In this present chapter we also anticipate a later chapter that introduces a new methodological innovation for connecting more evocatively with peoples' experiences (embodied interpretation). We conclude this chapter with some reflections on how this kind of research can lead humanly sensitive care.

Caring for a partner with Alzheimer's disease is a lived experience that is full of poignancy, steep learning, and complex coping. The intricate nuances of such a journey are beyond any words that try to characterise it. Qualitative research can however highlight important insights that may serve actionable knowledge (Van Manen, 1994) and practical wisdom (Polkinghorne, 2004).

In this present chapter we aim to generate a deeper understanding of six related phenomena within the intimate carer's journey that had been highlighted from a previous narrative study which focused on the breadth of the carer's journey (Galvin, Todres & Richardson, 2005). The previous study had characterised the journey as a whole, but generated the need to understand further a number of discrete phenomena within the journey in greater depth. Therefore, in the present study, each of these phenomena are considered complex enough to warrant an exploration of each of their structures in their own right (see Todres & Galvin, 2005, for a discussion of the relationship between narrative breadth and lifeworld depth). The present phenomenological study thus examines the structures of each of the following phenomena within the broader caring journey:

- Learning to live with the loved one's memory loss.
- The experience of adjusting to more limited horizons in their shared life together.
- Caring in practical ways.
- Adjusting to changes in the emotional relationship and level of intimacy.
- The transition to living apart.
- Advocating on the loved one's behalf.

Each of these themes carries complex challenges: to see a loved one change in this way; to leave behind what was and attend to what is now needed; to face issues of control, how much to 'take over' and how much to support a sense of personal agency and dignity; to lose the kind of reciprocity that couples work out in an intimate partnership; to face the limits of one's own caring abilities; to channel emotional energy into advocacy on behalf of 'this person who matters' within a complex system of care and processes.

Both the previous narrative study and the present phenomenological study were conducted by interviewing one carer (a husband, to be called Mark) on separate occasions about his experience of caring for his loved one (Marks's wife, to be called Lilly). The interview in the previous study was conducted in a way consistent with a narrative methodology. In the present study, an interview style consistent with the concern to elicit situated descriptions was adopted. Following from this, the chapter devotes itself exclusively to a presentation of findings from the phenomenological study. The advantage of concentrating on a single case study is that the researcher can focus on the seamless, internally related dimensions of such a complex experience. So, this is not a study about the range of unique variations that can occur for different carers. Nevertheless, there may be a kind of 'resonant' validity to the present study in that it highlights transferable possibilities for others in similar contexts.

Qualitative studies on caring generally, and caring for a loved one with Alzheimer's disease in particular, range from issues as general as 'presencing' and supporting (Beck, 2001; Chinn, 1991), comforting (Morse, 2000) and hope-giving (Farran, Herth & Popovich, 1995), to issues specific to caring for people with Alzheimer's disease, such as carers' changed understandings over time (Phinney, 2002), their concerns to advocate for the 'personhood' and dignity of the loved one (Ashworth & Ashworth, 2003) and their perceptions of the quality and nature of external care provision (Aggarwal et al., 2003).

The nature of reflective lifeworld research (Dahlberg, Dahlberg & Nystrom, 2008), of which this study is an example, is that the qualitative themes are often transferable beyond the particular phenomenon; so caring for people with Alzheimer's disease shares qualitative dimensions with that of caring in general. Different readers and audiences, in relation to their own area of interest or caring, may then reflect on those dimensions that are particular to caring for people with Alzheimer's disease and those that are related to caring in general. In this study, we are not aiming to be conclusive about the findings beyond their applicability to caring for people with Alzheimer's disease, but we leave this possibility open. The findings could be applied to a research project that attempts some form of systematic narrative review or qualitative metasynthesis of the carer's experience within a range of contexts (Jones, 2004; Finfgeld, 2003).

Methodological approach

To achieve detailed, concrete descriptions of each of the six phenomena (named above), a descriptive phenomenological research design was used (Giorgi, 1997; Giorgi & Giorgi, 2003a, 2003b; Giorgi 2009). The approach involved:

- Eliciting concrete, lifeworld descriptions for each of the delineated phenomena.
- Engaging in phenomenological analysis to explicate essential meanings by moving back and forth between the sense of the whole and its details.
- Arriving at a general, narrative description of each of the delineated phenomena (such findings are presented in this article as 'general structures').

We further modified this approach to communicate the findings in more evocative and empathic ways (Van Manen, 1994; Sells, Topor & Davidson, 2004), based on trying to complement the phenomenological rigour of Giorgi's 'scientific concern' with a 'communicative concern' (Todres & Holloway, 2004).

Todres (1998, 2000b) argued for the need to pay more attention to the aesthetic dimensions of phenomenological description and thus achieve both 'structure' and 'texture' in the way the findings of phenomenological research are communicated. Following other work by Todres (1999, 2004) that highlights the lived body's role in understanding meanings, we pursued the communication issue further by engaging in an additional phase of understanding and presentation that we called 'embodied interpretation'. In this way, we 'stand before' the general structures as 'embodied beings', and imagine in a bodily, grounded way what the general structures evoke and signify.

This embodied discipline is based on Gendlin's (1973) experiential phenomenology and the practice of 'focusing' (Gendlin, 1981). Whether to call this phase 'descriptive' or 'interpretive' phenomenology is a matter for debate. Van Manen (1994) sees a continuum between the two. Willis (2004) distinguishes a phenomenology that 'goes back to the things themselves' (scientific/validity concern) from a phenomenology that emphasises the question of 'what produces a feeling of understanding in the reader' (empathic/communicative concern). We take the view that a phenomenological study can do both, and that it may be useful to have a phase of presentation that is descriptive and one that is more interpretive. We also believe that it is still useful to distinguish these emphases, which is reflected in the presentation of this article.

Method

Mark, a carer for a loved one with Alzheimer's disease, approached us because he knew of our interest in doing this kind of research and wanted his experience to be of use to others. Mark's role was strictly that of informant who also gave feedback at the end as to the personal resonance and credibility of our descriptions and interpretation.

The issue here was not one of 'correspondence' with the details of what was said, but rather one of 'coherence' in relation to the sense and meaning of the communication.

A lifeworld-evoking question was initially asked about each of the six phenomena (Todres & Holloway, 2004). This was essentially a request for concrete descriptions of each of the phenomena as they were lived through. An example of such a question is: "Could you tell me about those times when you realised that a big change was happening in your social relationships with people?" The interview proceeded in a person-centred way, seeking clarification where necessary.

This interview phase was followed by the kind of analysis recommended by Giorgi and Giorgi (2003a). This analysis resulted in general structures of each of the six phenomena, which are first presented in a descriptive way in the findings section to follow. The main innovation to Giorgi's approach lies in a further phase of transforming each general structure into an 'embodied interpretation'. Each 'embodied interpretation' is thus presented after each general structure. In 'embodied interpretation', the phenomenologist's embodied self and 'digested understanding' becomes a locus of 'dwelling' with the meanings and allowing the described phenomenon to be 'let in'. This 'letting in' is enhanced further by being attentive to possible words, images and phrases that may be faithful to a *felt sense* of the understanding. It involves reading each descriptive general structure in this study a number of times, while being aware in a bodily way of what such empathic engagement feels like. It is an attempt to find the 'I in the Thou' (Buber, 1970) in that one finds a sense of common humanity in the resonance between us in relation to the phenomenon. These empathic understandings are therefore informed by the feelings in the body as well as the details in the text. This formulating process involves going back and forth between the general structure and the 'felt sense', waiting for a 'good enough' formulation that fulfils both the logic and details of the text as well as the bodily feeling of 'what it may be like'. This 'good enough' fit is an aesthetic recognition within the researcher. Mark was able to confirm that the 'embodied interpretations' were 'good words' that were consistent with his experience. There is some controversy whether this should be a criterion for validity, or whether the reader who reads a descriptive general structure followed by an 'embodied interpretation' is also well placed to assess whether the more evocative language of the 'embodied interpretation' carries forward the presented descriptive general structure in a way that also deepens the reader's empathic imagination and enlivens the phenomenon.

In this conception, 'validity' is not about 'correspondence' but about whether the embodied interpretation 'carries forward' the general structure in plausible and insightful ways. This means that such 'resonant validity' is 'always on the way' and never complete, because different readers apply the understandings to their own circumstances and concerns. Such a view of understanding is consistent with Gadamer's (1975/1997) notion of an 'application' rather than a unit of agreement.

Findings: General structures

A descriptive general structure of each of the six phenomena is followed in each case by the 'embodied interpretation' of that phenomenon.

Phenomenon 1: Learning to live with Lilly's memory loss

This kind of learning essentially involved coming to terms with how Mark's old expectations of Lilly's memory functioning no longer applied. This required the emotional learning of patience as well as a number of skills that would help Lilly.

The emotional learning of patience

Through numerous experiences of Lilly's memory loss, Mark first learned that he could not control or stop its exacerbation. Initially he found this extremely irritating and used the term 'nauseous' to express his visceral, angry, emotional reaction to what was, to him, the repetitiveness of her saying or doing something over and over again.

His initial angry response to her forgetfulness manifested itself in an attempt to control her into being less forgetful. This was part of his caring burden and at times he needed respite from it as his own health was suffering.

Coming to terms with Lilly's increasing memory loss involved a complex process of learning to be patient with her behaviour. This involved a number of observations and significant moments including the realisation that Lilly would become worse and unsettled in response to Mark's impatience. He became aware that his impatience produced a downward spiral in which Lilly would become further unsettled and confused; Mark would then feel remorse and wanted to avoid this in future.

Another key moment was when Mark saw that Lilly did not know how much her repetition was based on moment to moment memory loss. Once

Mark recognised this, he actively engaged in a process of testing and probing for what Lilly could and could not remember in particular circumstances. Previously he would have intervened, but later he learnt to let it take its course, if harmless. This helped him respond in a more patient and kindly way. He also learnt patience through a health professional, who helped him understand and normalise the nature of Lilly's memory loss and the implications for her behaviour, and through meeting other dementia sufferers at more advanced stages of memory loss.

Through this process of complex emotional, behavioural and cognitive learning, Mark developed some particular skills for responding to Lilly's memory loss that proved to be helpful, including:

- Validating and valuing activities just for their shared doing, rather than on the evaluation of the outcome. For example, helping Lilly occupy her time in unstructured moments.
- Kindly talking Lilly through her current situation that helped her know what to do next, such as encouraging her to actively participate in everyday tasks and prompting her to engage in routine and daily activities – skills such as eating that are necessary to sustain physical well-being.
- Using humour as a way to relieve his own tension and experience respite from his emotional discomfort in dealing with repetitiveness.

In summary, learning to respond to a loved one's memory loss involves an extremely challenging process; a letting go of previous expectations and the learning of a patient openness that does not take continuity for granted.

Embodied interpretation

To see a loved one change in this way. No! It is so natural to want to refuse that this is happening; that her memory can function as before. How deep is the urge to want to stop the exacerbation of memory loss in the loved one? It deserves at least an angry 'No', a great refusal, a denial in any way that is possible. At times, it is also a sinking feeling, the 'nausea' of an awareness that relentlessly breaks through. We *need* psychological strategies to temper the awareness that the memory loss cannot be stopped: anger towards self, loved one, professional. However, this is not enough to help, and helplessness, in this respect, dawns. It could be, as in Lilly's case, that a way of saying 'no' to the memory loss can affect the loved one in a negative way. She feels pressurised and upset. He feels remorse and such remorse also carries a dawning awareness that this way of trying to deny the memory loss does not work. It is ironic that the passionate 'no' to the memory loss is a care that can be experienced as a lack of care. As the intimate carer is able to 'let in', and accept to some degree, that the change is happening, care begins to take the form of patience. This is an evolving process, a hard-won spiral of insights and skills: awareness and acceptance of the loved one's changing limitations, actively testing out where the gaps are, learning from others who have gone before or can give guidance. But essentially the learning of patience is a shift from valuing outcome to valuing process. The intimate carer learns to 'hold back' from the need to rush to an outcome such as the successful completion of a task. Instead, he learns to 'be' with the process of 'what movement is possible' and of valuing this for its own sake; the mere moving of a piece in a puzzle, or beginning again a sentence from scratch. This kind of patience also involves 'holding' for the loved one that which she cannot hold: the holding of continuity. This kind of patience involves the challenging acceptance of discontinuity and the provision of continuity on the loved one's behalf.

Phenomenon 2: The experience of adjusting to more limited horizons

Mark is 'thrown into' a process of withdrawal from previous social horizons and simultaneously becomes engaged with more immediate preoccupations connected with the progression of Lilly's condition and the demands of being a carer.

There are two significant qualities to this experience. One is to do with the temporal reorganisation of expectations from what was a more possible future, to a now more limited future. The other is a social reorganisation.

The structure and qualities of temporal reorganisation

There was a growing realisation by Mark that he was being thrown into a situation that meant giving up a more active life, both for himself and in his shared life with Lilly. Within a short period, his life as a carer for Lilly became an urgent project and his time and energy were absorbed in the immediate concerns of care and advocacy. These more focused engagements were 'crowned' by signs of Lilly's physical deterioration and the coping challenges that this raised for them both. This was essentially a 'bitter pill' in terms of dashed hopes for the future and a realisation that renunciatory adjustments needed to be made to their long-term plans for life together.

Social reorganisation

There was a process of withdrawal from two kinds of social relationships. The first involved relationships that were more recent. In such circumstances, social opportunities lessened because of the unspoken discomfort experienced by all in the interaction, and also because of Mark's own preoccupation with the demands of caring and advocacy. This discomfort and social awkwardness occurred as a result of Lilly's changing mental condition.

Mark initially attempted to mediate and avoid the social discomfort and uneasiness in different ways, but described the following no-win situation:

- If he adopted a minimising or concealing approach to Lilly's condition, social awkwardness would occur as her condition became obvious.
- If, on the other hand, he was more open about it, he experienced a standoffishness. To Mark, others appeared to be uncomfortable and to want to have a metaphorical and real distance from the realities of dementia.

The second kind of social relationship involved old friends with whom they had a long history. These relationships were more comfortable for Mark and Lilly, and Mark believed that they were also more comfortable for their friends. Mark attributes this greater comfort to a joint history together, in which Lilly's surviving longer-term memory was more relevant than her short-term memory. In addition, these older friends were more willing and able to talk explicitly about Lilly's condition, which brought a greater degree of realism and acceptance to the social interaction.

Mark's experience of social awkwardness and discomfort made him sensitive to the way that people with Alzheimer's disease are stereotyped, stigmatised and distanced. Mark saw the withdrawal of others as a kind of self-protective defence against their own fears and concerns. Mark attempted to establish his own social network without Lilly, but a displacement of energy and preoccupation with caring hampered the possibility of meaningful, mutually-satisfying social encounters. Mark was left with a more introverted social life in which his more meaningful social relationships were at a distance.

In summary, Marks's social reorganisation involved the gradual loss of a meaningful and taken-for-granted social life in conjunction with an increasing engagement in the more immediate concerns of caring for Lilly. He also found he was increasingly sensitive to social discomfort from the problems of stigmatisation and stereotyping.

Embodied interpretation

To have your attention insistently called to the tasks of being a carer for a loved one with Alzheimer's disease – this is a strong pull, a renunciation, and a focused attunement to what now needs to be done. The loved one's condition becomes a pervasive consideration around which changing horizons become organised. This can be both a withdrawal from previous expectations and plans, and an increased concentration on the limitations of the changing circumstances and what is now possible. The 'strong pull' is the insistent 'what now' that calls; the demand for attention that the changing reality announces. The 'renunciation' is the letting go of what was previously important in the light of rapidly rearranging priorities. There is little time to mourn, as the readjustment requires attention. It is a more complicated kind of mourning than that of a sudden loss, where what is lost is clearer. The 'focused attunement to what now needs to be done' is not just about action but more importantly about the subtle tasks of finding the 'life that is possible' in the joint journey, the changes in the relationship and the challenges of care. It is a withdrawal from previous horizons and a concentration on 'this one': living with Alzheimer's disease, moment to moment, whatever the changing nature of this means as it unfolds. Time, with a future that was wide with more possibilities, becomes narrow. The task is then how to dwell and move from there. Old friends help. They remember a joint history and this is a sustaining resource through a changing story. Other social relationships may lose their ease and there may be a social renunciation that throws the carer and loved one more intensely together in a new way that requires adjustment. The loved one's carer is 'on call' and this poses the existential question of what kind of simple 'being together' is possible in the light of limited horizons.

Phenomenon 3: Caring engagement with changes in self-care behaviour and everyday routine

The context in which this form of caring engagement takes place is the gradual but significant deterioration of Lilly's short-term memory, in which taken-for-granted self-care, such as bathing, dressing, washing, routine and timing of appropriate activities, becomes increasingly disorientated.

Mark noticed how natural rhythms of light and dark, as reflected in seasons of the year, could exacerbate Lilly's disorientation of time and place. In such situations, Lilly would try to revert to previously established routines that did not fit the external situation. On the surface, this was manifested in what appeared to be untimely and inappropriate behaviour, such as not wanting to bathe, or wanting to get dressed at unusual times. More deeply, there was an initial and interpersonal struggle whereby her sense of agency and desire followed her internal sense of what was appropriate and timely, but which was different from Mark's more external orientation in terms of time and place.

Mark's caring engagement occurred on two levels. One, an implicit negotiation for agency, and two, explicit responsive and creative problem-solving strategies to address an increasing disorganisation in time and place, as manifested in self-care and routine activities.

The implicit negotiation for agency

Mark had to make ongoing assessments and judgements; when and where to remove the dilemma of agency and when not to. For example, in earlier stages of Lilly forgetting to bathe, Mark would prompt and remind her. However, in later stages this was ineffective and Lilly's feeling of agency in this matter was clearly important to her.

A creative strategy was used whereby Mark did not simply take control against Lilly's sense of what felt right to her. Through serendipity and creativity, Mark found a way to reframe the problem from self-care to that of a sharing and bonding experience. This worked to humanise the situation and achieve successful implicit negotiation of agency; turning 'you against me' into 'us'.

Creative problem-solving strategies

This was particularly important in the later stages of deterioration, when Lilly became more seriously disoriented about time and place, and when she accepted Mark's intervention to remove the dilemma of agency. This involved creative forms of practical problem-solving that developed in a common sense way in response to each new problem. For example, as Lilly's ability and timing for dressing herself deteriorated, Mark developed a series of strategies that responded to each level of difficulty. This ranged from labelling drawers and cupboards in the beginning, to leaving out clothing, and to physically dressing her. In the later stages, Lilly was quick to accept Mark's decisive and active intervention. Mark found that such decisiveness removed the dilemma of agency for Lilly and resulted in less argument and upset for both of them.

In summary, caring engagement with the loved one's changes in self-care ability and everyday routine involves a kind of care that humanises the transition from the struggle for personal agency to being a responsive caregiver who adapts to the different phases.

Embodied interpretation

To be in a dilemma about how much to 'take over' and how much to leave the loved one to her or his own devices; this is a complex concern, a 'care' that can result in 'too much' or 'too little'. Human dignity and the loved one's need to experience personal competence are at stake. The loved one with Alzheimer's disease wishes to assert a sense of personal identity that is intimately connected with a feeling of 'own-ness': 'my routine', 'my body', 'my privacy' – knowing what night means, knowing what day means, the rhythm of everyday life and the taken-for-granted habits of a lifetime. Into this coherent rhythm of own-ness comes disjunction. Meaningful links between body, mind, time and space begin to be interrupted. Therefore the intimate carer is called to hold continuity on behalf of the loved one. Here, the intimate carer may experience the acute dilemma of not wanting to take away the sense of personal agency and dignity that is possible. So he or she enters a changing process of 'negotiation' with the loved one; in a sense, 'asking for permission' to take over in areas that may require assistance. How do these issues of 'control' not obscure the experience of care? This is a very challenging existential question. Mark found ways in certain situations to humanise the 'taking over' by linking them with intimate sharing and bonding experiences – perhaps the sharing of a new diet or bathing together – where 'I' and 'you' can become 'we' or 'us'. In later stages of deterioration, the dilemma is less acute: the intimate carer may become less ambivalent about representing 'real-time continuity' and the loved one may be more ready to accept the intimate carer's intervention.

Phenomenon 4: Changes in emotional relationship and level of intimacy

The changes in their emotional relationship were characterised by three essential phases: a drifting apart, a complex and highly significant kind of reconnecting, and times of effortlessly being together.

Drifting apart

Both Lilly and Mark had difficulty accepting and coming to terms with this sense of drifting apart in their relationship. They had ceased to be 'man and wife' in an intimate and meaningful way and this was characterised by Mark as "just two people . . . putting up with each other". This sense of loss was experienced as yet another component of mourning. A further form of mourning involved having to readjust their previous aspirations for retirement and their view of the kind of life they would have had together: finding some way "to make the best of a very bad situation".

Reconnecting in a complex and significant way

Through a serendipitous event, Mark and Lilly found themselves in a situation characterised by a transitional quality between physical care-giving and physically intimate mutual relating. Previously, Mark had been exclusively focused on the physical care-giving demands of Lilly's condition. Following this event, Mark was able to reconnect with Lilly as a person, in a very simple, direct and tactile way, but which stopped short of full sexuality: they began showering together as an intimate way of solving bathing routine problems. This mixing of task and intimacy blurred the boundaries between instrumental care-giving and mutual relating. This new transitional quality proved to be a significant backdrop for regaining something that they once had, as well as for finding a new way of reincorporating this into the complex realities of changing roles.

These opportunities for physical intimacy continued and became more directly intimate (kissing and cuddling). Such moments of physical intimacy and 'skin to skin' contact also functioned as a background feeling that 'took the edge off' and broke through the struggles of control and resistance between them in their increasingly disparate and fixed roles.

Although these intimate physical interactions were not characterised by full sexuality, they were moments that Mark valued highly. These ties of intimacy were viewed as "the biggest and most monumental step forward other than drug therapy".

Effortlessly being together

Mark experienced a distinction between 'care-giving time' and simply 'being' with Lilly. Care-giving was often filled with instrumental tasks and strategies to help Lilly in routine and everyday tasks, and in helping her maintain a sense of continuity. The effortless flow of time could not just be taken for granted. Within the care-giving time, there were important 'pockets' of simply 'being' in which the flow of time became effortless. This was positively influenced by two kinds of support:

• An improved medication regime that helped Lilly's concentration so that they could enjoy each other's company more by simply being together.
• Increased support from a local health professional, who took the pressure off Mark and made him feel cared for. This gave him a sense of psychological respite, which helped him feel that he did not have to do everything or be on constant alert.

In summary, the way that Lilly and Mark were able to physically reconnect in a simple, tactile and unspoken way, provided the basis for a sustaining quality that saved the relationship from being merely functional.

Embodied interpretation

To lose the kinds of reciprocity that couples work out in an intimate partnership. The loved one inevitably becomes more dependent in many ways. The intimate carer becomes focused on more instrumental dimensions of caring for the loved one. This is a loss and constitutes a gap or 'hole' that emerges when simple, intimate partnership recedes. Such simple, intimate partnership may be longed for, as the instrumental challenges of care come to define the relationship more and more. There may be attempts at distraction by going away, or attempts at substitution by engaging in other activities. Still, the longing for simple intimate partnership may bubble in the background. The kind of intimate reconnection that is possible appears to be quite different from a reciprocal ongoing partnership of roles. It is less the project of partnership and more the possibility of simple moments of intimately being together. From project to moment – intimacy appears to be able to survive in the latter. Given the increasing 'brightness' of the emerging polarisation of roles (carer and cared-for), moments of simply 'being together' can break through. This is sometimes given in physical touch, or in silently sitting or walking together. This 'being' seems to require moments of unoccupied space and time. Ways of supporting such free moments of 'no consequence' are a great gift and help.

Phenomenon 5: The transition to living apart

For Mark, the timing of eventually living apart was not a decision that he actively took alone. Rather, he found his own health deteriorating and other professionals stepped in to suggest the need for living apart. Through this process he decided that the more time Lilly could spend in professional care, the better it would be for both of them. The way the separation occurred was important. Lilly moved to her care home for an initial respite break. After a period of being upset, Lilly appeared to adapt to the situation. Earlier experiences ('taster days') or brief separations appeared to help her settle to new living circumstances.

Mark was surprised to find that initially, during this respite, he did not miss her and experienced a relief at "not having to do anything". Through this initial trial separation, the adjustment to a more sustained living apart began. Mark's adjustment as a carer involved three forms of coping during the transition: circumstantial, emotional and meaning-making.

Circumstantial

Mark's own poor health at the time of their parting focused him initially on his own recovery process and he was forced to recognise the limits of his own caring capacity.

Emotional processing

Emotional processing involved the transition from guilt to reconciliation. After an experience of initial relief and respite, there was a period of feeling terribly guilty and a self-questioning about whether he had done the right thing. It was important and helpful for Mark that one of the health professionals (a community health nurse), "a person with trained good ears", functioned as an empathic and active listener to Mark's feelings of worry and guilt about the separation. He felt it was important and valuable to "pour out his inner soul" of having carried the burden. As part of this adjustment, it also helped him to see over time that the quality of the care Lilly received was good, and this reassured him. He felt grateful for this and characterised it as a "loving care" and "trusting care". Part of his emotional adjustment involved a cognitive reconciliation with the decisions that were taken. He came to feel that he had done the right thing compared with passively letting circumstances take their course.

Meaning-making

Already during the first 'trial' respite break, Mark began to think about how he could re-engage with his life in a different way. He had already begun to advocate on Lilly's behalf to ensure that she received the best medical treatment possible. After his own health recovered somewhat, Mark returned to an active life in which he could share the experience of caring for Lilly with others, and act on his strongly felt desire to raise awareness about Alzheimer's disease. This form of meaning-making and helping others has been successfully productive and gave him a sense of purpose. This busy life of meaningful advocacy helps Mark cope with what he experiences as the ongoing emotional challenge of missing their moments of intimacy and the effects of their separation. This emotional challenge has surfaced more in recent times as the busyness of his engagements recede. He is left with the challenge of how to occupy himself: "The worst thing for me is to be faced with having nothing to do."

In summary, the move to living apart has involved two central challenges: how to conscientiously accept and make sense of the separation, and how to live towards a different life of meaning, alone.

Embodied interpretation

To face the limits of one's own caring ability – how can this be resolved? Part of this emotional process involves experiencing a degree of helplessness in the face of unrelenting circumstances. The intimate carer may reach a time where he feels the intense burden of the caring tasks and the feeling of aloneness that sometimes comes with this. He would like to carry this burden; it is a care that he wishes to give. So there is often an inner resistance in the carer to the idea of living apart. The carer is painfully aware of the loved one's need for things to stay the same. In this case, the carer is conflicted about his own need for things to stay the same and the need for things to move on. There is a tragic awareness that their life together has come to this. It is extremely difficult for the carer to be deliberate in his decision to seek alternative living conditions for the loved one without her. When it happens, it is understandable that it may need to unfold in phases, with respite breaks and brief separations. Understandably, there can be guilt at times because 'who knows for sure' when a time of alternative living arrangements is necessary. It is an almost impossible decision to take alone, and the intimate carer may be greatly helped by another's listening ear. The intimate carer may even feel initially relieved if there is professional intervention to take the decision out of his or her hands. However, this sense of relief may be mixed with lonely self-questioning and further feelings of guilt. Some kind of justification of the separation helps to resolve this aspect of the parting to some extent. Such cognitive reconciliation can be partially achieved by seeing signs that some positive benefits have occurred in the quality of care that the loved one receives. It seems important for the intimate carer to see this and to experience such reassurance. When a degree of reconciliation to the parting has occurred, the intimate carer faces the challenge of another change of personal role: he or she becomes less instrumental in the care and this can open up the task of finding new meaning in a life alone. The other central challenge concerns what kind of 'visitor' the intimate carer becomes. There are inevitably a variety of responses to this question. Living apart is an accentuated 'fork in the road' and a 'saying goodbye' that comes and goes.

Phenomenon 6: Advocacy sustained by passion and know-how

By living through his complex experience of learning to care for Lilly, Mark developed both a passion and know-how that were demonstrated through his advocacy for Lilly in particular, and his concern to improve care for people with Alzheimer's disease in general. There were three kinds of advocacy that Mark actively engaged in:

- Representation, mediation and decision-making on Lilly's behalf.
- Raising awareness about neglected areas of concern in both the care and understanding of Alzheimer's.
- The passionate perseverance to be heard, and ensuring his advocacy made a difference.

Representation, mediation and decision-making on Lilly's behalf

Mark described a level of advocacy in which he acted as a mediator between Lilly's lived concerns and her difficulties in expressing these concerns during medical consultations. The need for this came not only from Mark's awareness of Lilly's lived difficulties in expression, but also from his awareness of the limited insights of professionals into the nuances of Lilly's problems. This was compounded by the bureaucratic/political constraints within which care options were offered. At times, the need for this form of mediation was felt by Mark to be urgent, and he would have to become 'extremely firm' in representing the perceived need. In this decision-making process, he had to consider Lilly's unique life and condition as a whole (for example, Lilly was also dealing with a malignant tumour).

The process of participating in this complex decision-making had to take into account Mark's understanding of Lilly's capacities and emotions, different professionals' advice, his knowledge of Lilly's idiosyncratic reactions to different medication regimes, and finally, his expectations about the kind of help and support they would get, both socially and medically.

Raising awareness of neglected areas of care

Beyond advocating specifically on Lilly's behalf, Mark became passionately aware of some general issues regarding the care of people with Alzheimer's disease. He wanted to raise awareness of these concerns within a broader public arena and share his own experiences, perspectives and expertise. Two specific concerns are incontinence care, and new and emerging drug regimes.

INCONTINENCE CARE

Mark has become aware of the extent to which incontinence care is a particular problem for males looking after females. He expresses empathy for other male carers in this situation and acknowledges his own privileged position whereby his background enabled him to cope. He feels that more can be done by health agencies to address these issues with specific reference to technical aids and medication.

NEW AND EMERGING DRUG REGIMES

Mark is concerned about how different agencies and professions compartmentalise the problems of caring for people with Alzheimer's disease, and he is strongly averse to those medical professionals who see the disease as primarily a social problem. In cynical moments, he wonders if this view is driven by cost considerations. He advocates strongly for new and improved drug regimes because he has noticed the significantly improved quality of life that Lilly has experienced since she started on new medication. He laments the fact that other sufferers may be deprived of this regime because of bureaucratic/political constraints, and lack of awareness and resources.

The passionate perseverance to be heard

A degree of perseverance, at different times, has been an important dimension for Mark in sustaining his advocacy. Such perseverance was indicated by seeking recourse beyond individual health care practitioners and agencies, to higher authorities that were responsible for political and executive decisions at different levels (for instance, Mark was prepared to seek legal recourse if necessary). This level of advocacy was fuelled by a number of experiences of not feeling heard in his mediation and advocacy role, and where simple negotiation in local situations did not appear to make a difference. There were some occasions in which he successfully achieved improvements in Lilly's treatment. As a consequence of his success in this higher level advocacy, Mark also achieved a sense of greater co-operation at the local level and began to feel cared for. He reflects on the need for a wider advocacy service.

In summary, this kind of advocacy was expressed as giving a voice to Lilly's needs from a perspective of *really knowing her*, perseverance in negotiating complex systems and a desire to influence the care of people Alzheimer's disease in general. This was driven by Mark's passion, prior experience, desire to share know-how and overriding concern for Lilly's wellbeing. The need to be heard and to make a difference in all these ways resulted in Mark experiencing some satisfying improvements.

Embodied interpretation

To take the gap, to want to go the extra mile – this may be the felt position of the intimate carer. Based on an unique knowledge of the loved one and on an intimate connection with 'this person who matters', there is an emotionally alive energy to want to enter any perceived neglected space between the needs of the loved one and the possible responses, either professional or situational, that might be available. How should the carer speak or act based on this emotional energy and unique knowledge? This may depend on personal style. In Mark's case, he drew on previous expertise in 'going the extra mile'. Others may find their own way of doing this. 'Taking the gap' can be a lonely responsibility and could become a burden. How to understand it and how to say it well to the right people may become a challenging preoccupation. In some cases, 'going the extra mile' may require perseverance in the face of others who may not yet understand the felt significance or importance of something the carer has seen or noticed. To be an intimate mediator between life with the loved one and the outside world is a steep learning curve. He learns a lot about what support and care is possible and available, and learns from 'within' about what is needed. The carer may become aware of how resources and help are part of a larger picture of health and social care services in general. The emotional energy to help make a difference may then exceed their particular situation, and the carer may join with others to advocate more generally on behalf of people experiencing the challenges of living with Alzheimer's disease. This could be as local as helping other carers, or as political as lobbying pressure groups for change. When done well, it could be a powerful form of advocacy, welcomed by relevant professionals and bodies. Whether just for them as a couple or for all sufferers, it appears important to the intimate carer to make a difference. So, knowing how to use this unique know-how and emotional energy is a core task for the intimate carer.

Implications and value of the study

We were asked to attend a local support group for carers' of people with Alzheimer's disease in order to communicate our findings of both the previous narrative study as well as this present phenomenological study. In responding to these findings, it emerged that each person (carer) in this group could relate personally the findings with particular unique nuances and variations. Each spoke further about differences or similarities, and each took the experience forward in different ways. We were happy with this because it served our concern not just to rest with the communication of 'propositional knowing', but how to turn this into the possibility of 'experiential knowing' (Heron, 1996; Reason, 1994a). Propositional knowing refers to general assertions that are abstract, such as 'a tranquilliser is good for anxiety'. Experiential knowing, on the other hand, goes further in that it relates the knowledge to our personal lives and experience; it allows us to see these experiences in a new light. Experiential knowing requires rich, evocative details to affirm personal meanings that have practical significance. This kind of phenomenological research includes attention to both the structural and textural, empathic, embodied dimensions, and we believe it possesses enough nuanced details to potentially turn propositional knowing into experiential knowing for readers.

Finally, we would like to close with some practice-related implications of this study by raising the following questions that focus on the carer's experience:

- How can professionals, family and support groups better recognise the 'irritation' and anger of carers as part of a *mourning* process that needs containment and help?
- How can professionals, family and support groups help the intimate carer to gradually move from valuing 'successful outcomes' of the loved one's memory and actions, to valuing 'process' for its own interactive sake and value?
- How can professionals become more aware of the practical wisdom in the intimate carer's remembrance of what is important to the loved one?
- How can professionals and support groups better understand, and respond to, the carer's struggle and dilemma of not wanting to take away the sense of personal agency and dignity from the loved one, while still managing the tasks of everyday routine and safety?
- How can professionals, family and support groups help the couple to have moments of 'simple being', where the instrumental role of the carer is relieved?
- When making the transition to living apart, how can professionals, family and support groups help the partner in the transition of role from 'intimate carer' to 'intimate visitor'?
- How can professionals, family and support groups help the carer find an appropriate level of advocacy that acknowledges his/her intimate knowledge while giving them permission to accept the limits of their caring abilities?

These questions all follow from the descriptive general structures generated from this study. Each question demonstrates the value of a phenomenological level of analysis that reveals specific experiential nuances that may also be transferable to other carers, such as: impatience as a resistance to mourning; how patience can be won by shifting from an emphasis on outcome to an emphasis on process; the intimate carer's important role in remembering what was important to the loved one; the dilemmas of caring for both the dignity and safety of the loved one; and a number of other important insights that are revealed by these descriptions. Readers can also imagine how some of these findings are generic and relevant to a range of caring situations beyond Alzheimer's.

An important question is, however, whether the 'embodied interpretations' added any value to the way the findings were presented. The rationale for this phase is to serve the communication of findings in more evocative ways that may support readers in understanding, what a phenomenon may be like, in an empathic way. The value of such empathic understanding is a kind of knowledge that is not so much about new

information (new contributions to propositional knowledge), but about the possibility of enhancing the emotional insight of audiences. This may be particularly important in the caring sciences where putting an experience together as an embodied whole may serve as an intuitive reference that can support acting in caring and ethical ways. In finding a way to be faithful to lifeworld descriptions, and expressing this in more evocative ways, the prose of 'embodied interpretations' may help to make an experiential phenomenon more present, so that it can live in ways that exceed any 'thin summary', and find a meaningful relationship with readers own lives: it is the kind of knowledge that 'touches'. The readers themselves may best judge the extent to which this works for them. Such 'resonant validity' was confirmed when we disseminated the findings presented in this chapter to a local support group for carers' mentioned previously. They were moved, and said that they wished for health professionals to understand these dimensions in such qualitatively rich terms.

Finally, we would like to suggest that by reading both the detailed information articulated in the descriptive structures as well as by reading the more 'evocative' sense of the 'embodied interpretations', fellow carers, professionals, family and support groups could be better equipped to understand and respond to the 'life that is possible' in this poignant journey. As one example of research-based knowledge for lifeworld-led care, this study may serve to indicate how finely textured descriptions from 'the insides' of 'what it is like' can offer fresh directions for a humanly sensitive practice.

Part II

Well-being and suffering
The focus of care

Part II points to the importance of understanding the experiential phenomena of well-being and suffering from a lifeworld perspective. We will show how a focus on well-being and suffering can give direction to care in important ways that are more complex than the narrower ideas of health and illness on their own. We will argue that these existential lifeworld phenomena of well-being and suffering crucially complement clinical and diagnostic categories, and as such, provide a necessary wider and deeper perspective from which the humanisation of care can be practised.

In Chapter 5 we offer an existential theory of well-being that is guided by Heidegger's later writings on 'homecoming'. We wish to show how such philosophical considerations can open up a productive way of thinking about 'what matters to people' and therefore to what human care could mean. We approach the question of what it is about the essence of well-being that makes all kinds of well-being possible. Consistent with a phenomenological approach, well-being is both a way of being-in-the-world, as well as a felt sense of what this is like as an experience. Drawing on Heidegger's notion of Gegnet (abiding expanse), we characterise the deepest possibility of existential well-being as 'dwelling-mobility'. This term indicates both the 'adventure' of being called into expansive existential possibilities, as well as 'being-at-home-with' what has been given. This deepest possibility of well-being carries with it a feeling of rootedness and flow, peace and possibility. However, we also consider how the separate notions of existential mobility and existential dwelling as discrete emphases can be developed to describe multiple variations of well-being possibilities.

In Chapter 6 we build on the existential theory of well-being, and offer a conceptual framework by which different kinds and levels of well-being can be named. As such, we provide a foundation for a resource-oriented approach in situations of illness and vulnerability (rather than a deficit-oriented approach). This alternative to a deficit-oriented approach is based on the critique that health and social care practices concentrate excessively on the 'clinical gaze' and as such, is an overly specialised focus that is too narrow. By means of a broader focus on the seamlessness of everyday life and its well-being possibilities, health care concerns may be meaningfully connected to more holistic conceptions of what is needed in humanly sensitive care. We then show how the existential theory of well-being can be further developed towards practice-relevant concerns. We introduce eighteen kinds of well-being that are intertwined and interrelated, and consider how each emphasis can lead to the formulation of resources that have the potential to give rise to well-being as a felt experience. We argue that, by focusing on a much wider range of well-being possibilities, practitioners may find new directions for care that are not just literal but that are also at an existential level.

But well-being is not enough. The experiences of well-being and suffering are in relation to one another: If care is to be humanly sensitive then practitioners require a view and understanding of both. Chapter 7 offers a conceptual framework by which different kinds and levels of suffering can be named. Various discourses have overemphasised well-being and obscured suffering, or overemphasised suffering and obscured well-being possibilities. Therefore, building on the previous chapters that articulated the philosophical foundations of the existential theory of well-being and which delineated eighteen kinds of well-being we now show how an 'existential theory of suffering' can underpin practice-relevant concerns. We introduce and name eighteen kinds of suffering that are intertwined and interrelated. This includes a descriptive vocabulary that goes beyond signs and symptoms and indicates the many ways in which the experience of suffering is seamlessly connected to all the aspects of an individual's life. We consider how each emphasis can lead to deeper understandings of what people may go through and offer 'a sensitising' framework for practitioners in such a way that they may be better equipped to offer forms of caring that do not exacerbate suffering. In other words, a meaningful understanding of the many dimensions of suffering provides a *capacity* for care, the subject of the forthcoming Part III of the book.

Chapter 8 provides an empirical illustration of well-being as 'Dwelling-mobility', drawing on a lifeworld study that describes older peoples' experiences of living in rural areas. The findings highlight what well-being means to older people, and underlines how well-being considerations are essentially transdisciplinary: health cannot be considered in isolation from other disciplinary concerns relevant to community life such as transport, heritage, technology and engagement in civic life. Although the study was initially designed to focus on the transport and mobility needs of older people living in rural areas, it soon became clear that these mobility issues could not be meaningfully understood without understanding their well-being priorities, the kinds of movement that constituted well-being, and how this related to the phenomenon of 'dwelling', which included their feeling of 'at-homeness' in their rural environment. But also, what emerged was a second phenomenon that we have called *rural living as a portal to well-being in older people*. The connection between well-being and rural place was constituted by two interrelated experiences: the importance of dwelling and slowing down in older age, and the importance of a 'rich textured locale' for the well-being of rural older people. We conclude this chapter by considering how the elders in our study may have something important to remind us: that mobility and sense of place are mutually implicated and that our present culture places an overemphasis on mobility, which may obscure the value of dwelling. More specifically, the illustration of older person issues is useful in highlighting how well-being is more than health: we show how resources and possibilities for well-being can be afforded even within the growing limitations of living as an ageing person within contemporary society.

5 An existential theory of well-being

'Dwelling-mobility'

In Chapter 3 we argued for a lifeworld-led care that could benefit from a focus on well-being as an important phenomenon in its own right. Building on the existential phenomenological tradition we began to offer a view of well-being as something much more than just the absence of illness. We have indicated how an articulation of what well-being is, is needed because it provides a positive understanding for the *direction* of care. Our view of well-being has been evolving, and this prompted us to dive deeply into this issue by going back to particular existential philosophical ideas. This chapter outlines these explorations and introduces our dwelling-mobility theory that is grounded in the ontological writings of Martin Heidegger:

> The proper dwelling plight lies in this, that mortals ever search anew for the essence of dwelling, that they *ever learn to dwell.*
> (Heidegger, 1993b, p. 363).

In this chapter we offer a theory of well-being that has been centrally informed by Heidegger's notion of 'homecoming'. We do not systematically present Heidegger's scholarly exposition and refer readers to other relevant texts (Heidegger, 1927/1962; 1966; 1971; 1973; 1993a; 1993b). Rather, we will draw on a particular aspect of Heidegger's later works in relation to homecoming and a particular development of this that he calls 'Gegnet'. We pursue the implications that these aspects of his work provide for an existential theory of well-being. This theory includes the notion of 'dwelling', the notion of 'mobility', and the unity of these two dimensions (Gegnet as 'abiding expanse'). More than providing a philosophical description of 'abiding expanse' we are particularly interested in how this possibility can be experienced by human beings as a great resource and possible direction.

Heidegger's task is philosophical and ontological. In relation to issues relevant to everyday human experience, he provides an ontological context; that is, he concerns himself with what it is about being-as-such that makes various kinds of human experiences possible. In other words, with reference to the phenomenon of human well-being, he provides a framework to approach the question: what is it about Being that gives to human beings the possibility of well-being? In drawing on Heidegger's later works we want to note the difference between his task as a philosopher and our task of trying to understand the implications of this ontological concern for well-being as a possibility in human life.

The specific trajectory of Heidegger's ontological writings that we wish to draw on concerns how his notion of homecoming can be usefully extended towards a more ontic understanding of the nature of well-being in our daily lives. We do this by building on Chapter 3 in which we articulated well-being as the intertwining of 'peace' and 'movement', at metaphorical, existential and literal levels. In articulating the essence of well-being, we also expressed these notions of peace and movement more metaphorically as 'home' and 'adventure'. Here, we wish to expand our earlier notion of peace towards the more encompassing term 'dwelling' and expand our earlier notion of movement towards the more encompassing term 'mobility'. More than this, we will consider how Heidegger's notion of 'Gegnet' can open up an understanding of how 'dwelling' and 'mobility' are both implicit in the deepest experience of well-being. We are substantially guided in this trajectory by Mugerauer's (2008) book *Heidegger and Homecoming*, but wish to use his analysis in a way that can throw some light on the phenomenon of human well-being. Mugerauer helped us to see how a rather obscure idea in Heidegger's work, namely 'Gegnet', could be highly productive when trying to integrate the experiences of movement and stillness.

The discourse that is especially relevant to well-being occurs in a number of Heidegger's later works (1966; 1971; 1973; 1993a; 1993b). In some of these texts he describes the 'togetherness' of things in an interrelated horizon that gives space for things and their movement ('the four fold' of sky, earth, mortals and divinities). This 'together' four fold is the source for the possibility of dwelling with things as they are, and moving with things as they become what they can. It is this ontological 'togetherness', with its 'horizon' of room-making (einraumen), that provides the template within which human beings' experience of 'dwelling with', and 'moving with', can be credibly understood.

The ontological possibility of well-being: The harmony of dwelling and mobility

Heidegger's (1993a, 1993b) introduction of the four fold (sky, earth, mortals and divinities) is his way of indicating an alternative ontological context for the relationship between Being and beings, an alternative to the technological perspective of the Western metaphysical tradition. The Western metaphysical tradition posits neutral space within which one can 'put' beings and things, and time is the neutral context in which all things happen sequentially. But Heidegger was concerned that this metaphysical framework missed a 'cosmos' in which Being was not just space and time (merely a neutral context), but a wholeness that was more intimately implicated in the way beings are related to one another and Being-as-a-whole. This relatedness is both a relatedness of movement and a relatedness of kinship and is indicated in Heidegger's (1966) notion of Gegnet.

Gegnet gives both a continuity between Being and beings, as well as a rupture, so that beings can become figural and stand out of their ground. Gegnet means open expanse or abiding expanse, but it is at the same time also a gathering. 'The gathering is a multidimensional letting' (Mugerauer, 2008, p. 467).

Human beings are intimately implicated in Gegnet by being the 'there' of being, the 'place' where there is a clearing for the gatherings of beings and things; in this way being-as-such does not happen without human being.

Heidegger then also offers a consideration of how this ontological context above can be relevant for the ontic everyday lives of human beings. Can a human being remember his or her own dwelling in Being while also sojourning in the 'mobility-current' of being, thus called into a novel future? We would like to leave this ontological analysis for now, and consider how this framework may play out in relation to the human experience of well-being.

Delineating the phenomenon of human well-being

In his book *The Hermeneutics of Medicine and the Phenomenology of Health*, Svenaeus (2000) draws on Heidegger's (1927/1962) *Being and Time* and the 'Zollikon Seminars' (Heidegger, 2001) to progress a view of health as 'home-like being-in-the world': "Health is to be understood as a being-at-home that keeps the not-being-at-home in the world from becoming apparent" (Svenaeus, 2000, p. 93). In this present chapter we cannot do justice to all the ways that Svenaeus insightfully elaborates this theme. However, building on some of these insights we would like to concentrate more on how the phenomenon of 'homelessness', although never fully eradicated, can become reframed within a more encompassing possibility of homecoming: the possibility of finding home within the homeless.

The journey through homelessness before authentic homecoming

In *Being and Time* Heidegger refers to a form of being-at-home (zuhause) that is inauthentic in that human beings can take excessive refuge in 'das man' or 'the man-in-general'. Such taken for granted familiarity constitutes a kind of 'at-homeness' but at great cost to what he sees as the possibility of taking on a life of one's own. The numbing comfort of this taken for granted familiarity is in Heidegger's view not sustainable, as human finitude and vulnerability inevitably announce themselves in many ways. In his analysis of the journey towards authenticity, he emphasises the importance of anxiety as a form of attunement that opens up a certain aloneness in facing the uncertain cares of one's personal life that is always in the shadow of its potential falling away. Heidegger uses the term 'uncanniness' (unheimleich) to indicate this kind of existential homelessness that is faced when one is able to embrace the 'resolute' responsibility of moving away from the 'taken for granted' securities of the familiar 'at-homeness'. Within this perspective, ill health can be one of the ways in which human vulnerability reminds us of an existential homelessness that cannot be denied. Illness then can be 'a wake-up call' to face existential tasks that may have been avoided. If Heidegger just left us here he would leave us in quite a nihilistic position in which we have to stoically come to terms with our homelessness. But later, in what Mugerauer (2008) calls 'the homey papers' Heidegger articulates another kind of homecoming that is authentically possible for human beings: a movement from the inauthenticity of a familiar being-at-home (zuhause) through a more authentic embrace of existential homelessness to the possibility of an authentic homecoming. Facing this 'not being at home', although an anxiety provoking experience, can also open up a path of movement; and this can provide an energising potential that can itself be felt as well-being. Homelessness paradoxically provides an important motivation for the quest to seek the experience of homecoming. Our theory of well-being thus wishes to incorporate the value of experiences of homelessness as well as experiences of homecoming. As will be shown, homelessness gives mobility to life as a positive potential, while homecoming gives peace to life as a positive potential.

An existential theory of well-being as 'dwelling-mobility'

The following exposition of our existential theory of well-being first articulates existential mobility and existential dwelling as distinct dimensions before considering them together, and dialectically, as the unity of dwelling-mobility.

Existential mobility

In many different ways Heidegger conveyed how homelessness does not just bring insecurity, but also provides the ontological possibilities of authentic movement or what we call 'existential mobility'. Homelessness carries with it a sense of unfinishedness that seeks future possibilities, people and projects. It is a creative restlessness in which we are called into our future possibilities. We could say that it is a kind of 'eros' or energy which can give a feeling of flow, aliveness and vibrant movement. When called in this way we may feel connected to our life's desires. We can also metaphorise this movement as a 'sense of adventure'. Therefore such existential mobility forms one of the dimensions of our theory of well-being.

Although they do not use this term, it could be said that the writings of Boss (1979), Gadamer (1996) and Toombs (1993) emphasise this notion of existential mobility in their considerations of well-being. In this view, well-being is about the access to one's existential possibilities in time and space, with one's body and with others. In emphasising the notion of possibilities, we are also emphasising the 'forward moving' quality of living towards the future and finding meaningful projects there. For Boss (1979), well-being is understood as all the ways in which we are able to have access to, and actualise a full range of experiential and behavioural possibilities as articulated by Heidegger in *Being and Time*. These possibilities, which Heidegger called 'existentiale', include spatiality, temporality, intersubjectivity, embodiment, and mood. For Boss, to restore well-being is to restore one's potential to be connected in all of these ways. Thus for example, to help restore a depressed person's temporal range, the psychotherapist becomes interested in the ways in which the future has become uninviting to the person; to help restore well-being for a person whose physical movement is very limited, a helper may focus on the well-being possibilities of facilitating contact with greater spatial horizons through accessing beautiful and expansive sights, smells and sounds; to help restore well-being in an ill person isolated in intensive care, a mere human touch or voice may be the intersubjective welcome that is needed to invite the person out of their sense of isolation. In his writings on health and well-being, Gadamer (1996) indicated how healthy people are embodied in such a way that they are un-preoccupied with their physical condition, thus free to participate in all the powers that their bodies afford. Also, Toombs (1993) provides a number of descriptions of ill health as the truncation of, or deficit in, healthy existential possibilities of spatiality, temporality, intersubjectivity, embodiment and mood. Both Heidegger and Boss have emphasised how these different existential possibilities are equi-primordial, that is, that they are all implicated in one another without privileging any one of them in a way, which sets up any particular existential dimension as primary. Our theory of well-being, in its emphasis on 'existential mobility', is thus interested in all of the ways one can experience existential mobility with different emphases. However, this dimension of 'existential mobility' alone is at risk of obscuring another equally important but distinctive dimension of well-being: the dimension that we call 'existential dwelling'.

Existential dwelling

In his later work Heidegger became more focused on a kind of existential homecoming that authentically grounds the human potentiality for a peaceful attunement to existence. In his writings on 'letting-be-ness' (Gelassenheit), and 'making a space for', Heidegger articulated the possibility of a human relationship to being that was characterised by acceptance and the possibility of peace. Already in *Being and Time* there was a concern to face and come to terms with finitude and the existential vulnerabilities of existence. There is some question here about the extent to which such 'coming to terms' was a true acceptance rather than a resolute form of courage to bear one's alone-ness and responsibility. After what has been called the 'turning' (Kehre), Heidegger concerns himself much more directly with the kind of comportment required that allows Being and beings 'to be'. He believed that this had great import for a philosophical project that tries to think Being in a fresh way that is more original than traditional Western Metaphysical frameworks.

However, implicit in this we also find some important clues for a more peaceful attunement to life's everyday vicissitudes. In the comportment of 'Gelassenheit' or 'letting-be-ness' there is an openness to allow whatever is there to simply be present in the manner that it is present, before one rushes in to try to change it. We would like to express the essence of this quality in the term 'existential dwelling'. To dwell is to come home to one's situation, to hear what is there, to abide, to linger and to be gathered there with what belongs there. When such dwelling is able to be fully supported, there may be a mood of peacefulness. But peacefulness is only one possible attunement within dwelling. The essence of dwelling is simply the willingness to be there, whatever this 'being there' is like. One can come to dwelling in many ways such as sadness, suffering, concern, attentiveness, acceptance, relaxation or patience. Dwelling is intentional in its attunement in that it allows the world, the body, things, others and the flow of time to be what it is. It is a form of being grounded in the present moment, supported by a past that is arriving and the openness of a future that is calling. Dwelling makes room for all this. Although peacefulness and 'being at one' with 'what is there' is its deepest calling and possibility, such homecoming is invariably through homelessness if it is to be authentic. To dwell is to 'come home' to what is there with oneself and the world, whatever the qualities of that may be.

There is a paradox to existential dwelling. In coming home to what 'is there', there is not necessarily an eradication of suffering, pain and the existential vicissitudes of life. So how can such dwelling constitute a core dimension of well-being? What is it about this dwelling that can be called well-being? Just this: that there is a felt quality to 'making room for' and 'letting-be-ness' that constitutes a kind of peace, in spite of everything, that is different from the kind of peace that depends on the eradication of limiting conditions. If we were to follow Heidegger's project to speak the possibility of possibilities, we would say that, in existential dwelling, human being is inhering in Being; that is, that such dwelling is not just a psychological state but a description of a relationship of belonging between human being and her/ his ground.

Conceptually it is possible to distinguish the two dimensions of mobility and dwelling: mobility emphasises the call of the future and the energetic feeling of possibility; dwelling emphasises a settling into the present moment with its acceptance of things as they are. In his later work however, Heidegger opened up the term 'Gegnet', and offers a way to speak of how dwelling and mobility can come together as an integrated unified experience that forms the deepest possibility of well-being. We thus now turn to Gegnet and what we have called 'dwelling-mobility'.

Dwelling-mobility: Gegnet

In this section we wish to consider how Heidegger's notion of Gegnet may help us to think about the ultimate essential unity of mobility and dwelling in the context of well-being.

Heidegger never eradicates the givenness of homelessness, but what he does open up at various levels and stages is a space in which homelessness does not exclude the possibility of well-being. This kind of well-being has to be inclusive enough in order to hold open the possibility of homecoming within homelessness. He thus had to find a language and a way of thinking that could express this paradox. Because the words 'dwelling' and 'mobility', 'home' and 'homelessness' divert attention from each other, it is difficult to imagine how both these dimensions can live together as a source of well-being. But we can do this by unfolding some of the implications of Heidegger's use of the term Gegnet in an ontological context. Mugerauer (2008) provides a useful summary of what is meant by the term:

> Gegnet is the opening that lets the horizon come forth as horizon, permits all to shelter, and lets everything come back home to its ownness, which is, at one and the same time, in/ as their belonging together. *To the already potent figure of homecoming in 'return to itself', Heidegger adds the long-anticipated, long held off final possibility of completion: opening gathers and returns everything 'to rest in its own abiding' to rest, to stay at home in itself and to that to which it belongs.*
>
> (Mugerauer, 2008, p. 467, original italics).

Implicit in this idea of Gegnet as 'gathering in the abiding expanse' is a sense in which there is both the freedom and openness of mobility (being called into the novelty of open horizons) as well as the 'coming back home to itself' of dwelling (resting in the peacefulness of its own abiding). This togetherness of mobility and dwelling provides the possibility of well-being with both a 'rootedness' as well as a 'flow'. This rooted flow, this 'dwelling-mobility', is a space in which 'homecoming' can be found by embracing 'homelessness'. So in Gegnet there is always already the togetherness of dwelling and mobility. To sojourn in 'dwelling-mobility' is to . . . 'endure in the abiding expanse' (Mugerauer, 2008, p. 469).

Summary of existential theory of well-being: Dwelling-mobility

In this theory we approached the question of what it is about well-being that makes all kinds of well-being possible. Thus our phenomenon is about the structure of well-being before any particular categorisation of well-being, such as, for example, physical well-being, social well-being, emotional well-being, economic well-being. Our structure of well-being thus makes these categorical forms of well-being possible and provides the essence of well-being that coheres through all its variations.

Consistent with a phenomenological approach, well-being is both a way of being-in-the-world, as well as how this way of being-in the-world is felt as an experience.

The deepest possibility of existential well-being lies in the unity of dwelling-mobility. Guided by Heidegger's notion of Gegnet, dwelling-mobility describes both the 'adventure' of being called into existential possibilities as well as the 'being at home with' what has been given. This deepest possibility carries with it a feeling of rootedness and flow, peace and possibility.

However, the variations of well-being lie in the dialectic of mobility and dwelling, as well as the relative emphasis that each dimension offers as a possible variation of well-being.

The essence of mobility lies in all the ways in which we are called into the existential possibilities of moving forward with time, space, others, mood and our bodies. The feeling of this 'moving forward' is one of energised flow.

The essence of dwelling lies in all the ways that we existentially 'come home' to what we have been given in time, space, others, mood and our bodies. The feeling of this 'coming home' is one of acceptance, 'rootedness' and peace.

Well-being, as we have articulated it, is a positive possibility that is independent of health and illness but is a resource for both. In other words, well-being can be found within illness and well-being is more than health. However, we wish to acknowledge that well-being, as an ontic everyday experience, is never complete, but something of the essence of well-being provides a possibility that always calls and can shine through. As such, our theory of well-being as 'dwelling-mobility' describes a capacity for movement and a capacity for settling.

Well-being possibilities: Kinds and levels of well-being

Gegnet as an experiential possibility is inclusive of all the kinds and levels of well-being. It would appear to be an existential possibility that calls to us from deep within embodied being. In a sense, the body knows this unity of dwelling-mobility, even though one's life circumstances and conscious experience may not often present this deepest possibility of well-being. However the emphases that we have articulated as mobility and dwelling can also provide a conceptual foundation for considering various levels and kinds of well-being that stop short of the unity of dwelling-mobility. We would like to offer several kinds of well-being experiences in which dwelling and mobility occur with a number of different emphases. These emphases are informed by the following lifeworld constituents as articulated by Husserl and elaborated by Heidegger: spatiality, temporality, intersubjectivity, mood and embodiment. When dwelling is experienced in a spatial way one has a sense of being at home; when mobility is experienced in a spatial way one has a sense of adventure. When dwelling is experienced in a temporal way there is a sense of being grounded in the present moment; when mobility is experienced in a temporal way there is a sense of temporal 'flow' and forward movement. When dwelling is experienced in an intersubjective way there is a sense of kinship and belonging; when mobility is experienced in an intersubjective way there is a sense of mysterious interpersonal attraction. When dwelling is experienced as mood there is a sense of peace; when mobility is experienced as mood there is a sense of excitement or desire. When dwelling is experienced as a form of personal identity there is a sense of being at 'one with' the world; when mobility is experienced as a form of personal identity there is sense of 'I can'. When dwelling is experienced in an embodied way there is a sense of comfort; when mobility is experienced in an embodied way there is a sense of vitality.

All these experiential qualities, although overlapping, provide distinctive nuances or emphases. As such they can provide a conceptual framework for the range of distinctive resources that can be drawn upon or developed on in peoples' well-being journeys.

If one was trying to take this framework into a more applied direction one would be concerned with facilitating possibilities for 'movement' as well as possibilities for 'letting-be-ness' at both existential and literal levels.

We develop this framework further in the next chapter, and indicate some of the implications of this framework for practice. The practical applications, however, proceed from a thoughtfulness about different kinds of mobility and dwelling at literal, metaphorical and existential levels, and how these different possible variations may be experienced within the context of fundamental lifeworld structures ('existentiale') such as temporality, intersubjectivity, embodiment, spatiality and mood. This *sensitising* (rather than prescriptive) way to consider the kind and level of well-being that may be possible in a concrete circumstance may offer some practical directions which we illustrate in greater depth in Chapter 6. But for now, informed by the theory, one may think of one kind of possible well-being variation as 'spatial mobility', another as 'temporal mobility', and another as 'mooded dwelling', etc. In thinking about the question of what spatial mobility is possible for a person, one could, together with a person who has complex disabilities, and can't go outside, consider what expansive spatial horizons may be possible within that context. An example of 'temporal mobility' may refer to the challenge of how to help a person access past memories (move into the past) when their short-term memory is failing. An example of 'mooded dwelling' may refer to the challenge of how to help a person feel more peaceful and 'at home' in a busy clinical care environment.

So, the theory itself may begin to provide a way of thinking about what the ontic possibilities and variations of well-being could be within the ontology of well-being as a human possibility.

Within this perspective of well-being, people find their own unique way towards well-being, and there is a play between all these nuances, one's personal history, and the limitations that life presents. But in all these variations, the body knows something about well-being as 'dwelling-mobility', and such tacit knowing forms the experiential touchstone for guiding our quest towards homecoming within the homeless.

6 Kinds of well-being

Eighteen directions for caring

As previously indicated, a lifeworld-led approach to care does not only provide an alternative descriptive power, but also a directional power, given by a consideration of well-being. If well-being offers a core direction for caring then it is important to begin to articulate adequate conceptualisations of well-being that can do justice to both the essence of what it is, and to its possible variations in human lives. It is for this reason that we have found it highly productive to draw on a phenomenological style of philosophy in order to offer a conceptual framework that can articulate a multiplicity of kinds of well-being, and some of the possible paths towards it. But let us start with well-being as an intertwined experiential phenomenon.

Our bodies know what well-being is.[1] We recognise well-being in many different forms and nuances when it is present, and recognise its absence in suffering. When asked the question 'how are you?', if we take a moment, as human beings, we can sense very concretely our state of well-being or otherwise, even if we are not able to find the best words to say all of it. This experiential sense of well-being can be articulated in many different ways. In the previous chapter we asked the question: What is it about the essence of well-being that makes all kinds of well-being possible? There, we articulated the deepest experience of well-being as a unity of dwelling and mobility. We indicated how our well-being theory was inspired by a particular interpretation of Heidegger (Mugerauer, 2008), an interpretation that considers the trajectory of Heidegger's work as a whole including both the continuities and discontinuities of his earlier and later works. This interpretation was central to our more applied concerns about the phenomenon of well-being.[2]

---

1 We cannot here pursue the continental philosophical reasoning behind this statement. Suffice to say that we do not just mean simply 'subjective well-being', but rather an understanding that is based on Heidegger's "Befindlichkeit" and further pursued in Merleau-Ponty's ideas. Here, experiential well-being is seen as a bodily informed phenomenon that speaks of our relation to Being. That is, it is an intentional bodily phenomenon that can tell us something about ways of living in the world.

2 There are many different interpretations of Heidegger and the controversies concerning his earlier and later works. However in following Mugerauer, we have been encouraged by finding similar broad interpretations of Heidegger in other scholars such as Safranski (1999), Inwood (1999) and Moran (2000).

Here we also followed in the '*Zollikon Seminars*' (Heidegger, 2001) in which an ontological level of analysis is seen to have important potentially practical ontic insights for our everyday lives. It is in this spirit that we have attempted to translate these ideas into its consequences for understanding human well-being and the practical implications this may have for caring.

A typology of well-being

In our previous chapter, we indicated that the unity of dwelling-mobility has within it a sense of both mobility and dwelling.[3] Thus experiences of possibility and peace, flow and rootedness are not necessarily separate experiences even though they may be articulated as logically discrete. The nature of embodied experience is that it is able to hold multiple qualities at the same time. This unity of dwelling-mobility indicates well-being in its deepest fullness, but does not have to be experienced in this fullest sense to be of benefit to people: there can be different kinds and levels of well-being that can be derived from this unity, depending on emphasis and focus. It is in this spirit that we have derived eighteen variations of well-being experience. In Table 6.1, we introduce what we call 'the Dwelling-Mobility Lattice'.

An explanation of this framework

On the left hand side of Table 6.1 we name a number of experiential domains within which well-being can be emphasised (spatiality, temporality, etc.). These experiential domains are centrally informed by the phenomenological-philosophical tradition in which Husserl, Heidegger, Merleau-Ponty and others have delineated fundamental lifeworld constituents that are implicated in human experience (Boss, 1979; Heidegger, 1927/1962; Husserl, 1936/1970; Merleau Ponty, 1945/1962).[4] So for example, one can think of well-being in terms of the way it can be experienced spatially, temporally, interpersonally, bodily, in mood, and in terms of the experience of personal identity. Although each of these domains of experience are implicated in one another, one can still usefully refer to these qualities as emphases, and this

---

3 Previously, we have indicated that in *Being and Time* although homelessness is more profound than 'at-homeness', in Heidegger's later work (particularly *Building, Dwelling and Thinking*; *Art and Space* and [Gelassenheit] *Discourse on Thinking*), he emphasises at-homeness more and more, even though this never eradicates homelessness, and we thus ended the previous chapter with how Heidegger raises the possibility of homecoming within the homeless.

4 We acknowledge that these philosophers do not necessarily agree about the nature of these experiential domains and the differential roles that they play. In this respect, we mainly follow Heidegger and Boss in naming these domains but, following Merleau-Ponty (1945/1962) and Ashworth (2003), on the notion of 'self-hood', we have found it useful to add the dimension we call 'identity' as it provides a helpful nuance to our theory of well-being.

Table 6.1 'Dwelling-mobility' lattice

	MOBILITY	DWELLING	DWELLING-MOBILITY
SPATIALITY	Adventurous horizons	At-homeness	Abiding expanse
TEMPORALITY	Future orientation	Present centredness	Renewal
INTER-SUBJECTIVITY	Mysterious interpersonal attraction	Kinship and belonging	Mutual complementarity
MOOD	Excitement or desire	Peacefulness	Mirror-like multidimensional fullness
IDENTITY	I can	I am	Layered continuity
EMBODIMENT	Vitality	Comfort	Grounded vibrancy

can help us to delineate different well-being possibilities. Along the horizontal rows, the two emphases of well-being (dwelling and mobility) are delineated, together with a third possibility when intertwined or unified (dwelling-mobility). Indeed, ontologically, this intertwined phenomenon is primary and the separate emphases of dwelling and mobility are variations that exist in 'stepped down' ways ('figure/ground' emphases within a unity). So, considering each of the qualities of well-being as both separate and intertwined (dwelling, mobility, the unity of dwelling-mobility), one can see these qualities more clearly as a 'structure' with different emphases or variations in everyday life. For example, one can think of a well-being possibility where mobility is emphasised, a well-being possibility where dwelling is emphasised, and a well-being possibility where they are integrated. By considering the relative interaction of these two dimensions (experiential domains and well-being possibilities) one can derive a number of kinds and levels of well-being that are afforded to human existence. In this framework we have derived eighteen terms that each describe a particular quality of well-being such as 'present-centredness' when dwelling and temporality interact, or 'I can' when identity and mobility interact.

Although these variations are all implicated in one another, their distinct experiential emphases in terms of figure and ground can be usefully delineated and named. For example, one may experience a kind of well-being in which spatial dwelling is in the foreground; here, one may feel particularly tuned into the physical environment's quality that engenders a sense of 'at-homeness' as a foreground experience. This emphasis is 'never alone' or apart from other possible well-being variations. So the mood of dwelling (that has a quality of 'peacefulness') may also be there, but in the background, and not explicitly focused upon. Nevertheless, we will now show that it is helpful to articulate each of the variations of well-being as discrete emphases. We call this framework a 'lattice' because the various kinds of well-being are dynamically intertwined and layered. The term 'lattice' attempts to indicate this woven nature and to express the dynamic possibilities of their figure/ground relationships within their larger unity. We now describe each variation of well-being experience. We believe that these discrete emphases are both experientially meaningful, as well as having value when one comes to think about practical directions. Furthermore, to make comparisons between the eighteen variations of well-being, we address similar topics within each variation. Although this may appear formulaic and perhaps repetitive to read, we do this for the sake of rigour and to be able to show how the various elements are similar or different across variations. So in each case, we consider how that dimension is essentially defined, give an example of how it may be lived, provide a possible health care application, etc.

Spatial mobility: Adventurous horizons

There is a well-being experience that emphasises 'adventurous horizons'. When adventurous horizons are bright, a person is tuned into the spatial possibilities of their environment that offer movement (either metaphorically or literally) in ways that are valued or wanted. So for example, a sense of adventurous horizons in a literal sense may occur 'on the road' where one feels invited to explore new places and things; there is a 'sense of adventure' provided by the spatial possibilities of the situation. A sense of 'adventurous horizons' in a metaphorical way may occur through, for example, reading a novel in which descriptions of place open up a feeling of adventure as imagined movement.

In relation to the implications of this 'well-being emphasis' for care, one could ask the question: what adventurous horizons in this person's physical environment can be offered and supported as either a literal reality or as a focus for possible experiential engagement? One example of offering adventurous horizons as a possible experiential focus that is not literal may occur in the case of a person who is physically disabled. Here, some time may be spent in which carers find out about the kind of imaginative journeys that could be meaningful to a person, and engage in help that could open up such a possibility either through access to paintings, or films and so on. Alternatively, literal possibilities may include outings that achieve something of the essence of this felt sense in a way that is possible. Another example might simply be the sense of adventurous horizon in which a person experiences the feeling of spatial mobility by looking out at the stars or a sunset. Well-being as a sense of 'adventurous horizons' is thus anything that offers a place of promise.

Spatial dwelling: At-homeness

There is a well-being experience that emphasises 'at-homeness' or a sense of 'being at home'. When there is a sense of 'being at home' a person may be tuned into the spatial possibilities of their environment that offer settling or stillness (either metaphorically or literally) in ways that are valued or wanted. So for example, a sense of at-homeness in a literal sense may occur 'on my favourite easy chair in front of the fire'. Here, literally, one is in physical surroundings that are familiar and comfortable; there is a sense of at-homeness provided by the spatial possibilities of the situation. A sense of at-homeness in a metaphorical sense may occur through, for example, having familiar objects and personal things close to hand, that connect a person to their familiar sense of place and belonging; this returns one spatially to a sense of at-homeness as an experience of welcome 'dwelling'. In relation to the implications of this 'well-being emphasis' for care, one could ask the question: what sense of 'at-homeness' in this person's physical environment can be offered and supported as either a literal reality or as a focus for possible experiential engagement? One example of offering welcome 'at-homeness' as a possible experiential focus that is not literal might be where a person is being treated in a clinical environment. Here, there is a danger that the person may feel dislocated or alien, and some effort may be spent bringing in objects and things into the environment that provide a sense of familiarity and belonging. This could range from plants and other natural items to personally significant objects that connect the person with their familiar sense of place. Well-being as a sense of at-homeness is anything that offers a place of settling or peace.

Spatial dwelling-mobility: Abiding expanse

There is a well-being experience that can hold both spatial mobility and spatial dwelling together; an experience that can straddle both adventurous horizons and at-homeness. We call this experience 'abiding expanse'. In 'abiding expanse', a person is tuned into the spatial possibilities of their environment that offers at the same time 'settled at-homeness' as well as 'adventurous horizons', either metaphorically or literally in ways that are valued or wanted. In this unity, there is an experience of abiding expanse; being deeply connected to a familiar place that offers itself as a stepping out point for possible literal or metaphorical adventures or journeys. So, for example, one person may have a sense of abiding expanse, in both literal and metaphorical ways, at a window where he or she feels both safe and settled inside, as well as invited out by the path disappearing into the distance. In relation to the implications of this well-being emphasis for care, one could ask the question: What possibilities of 'abiding expanse' can be offered in this person's physical environment and supported as either a literal reality or as a focus for possible experiential engagement?

One example of facilitating 'abiding expanse' as a possible experiential focus is where a person is physically disabled. Here, instead of just facilitating imaginative journeys in different ways or bringing familiar objects into the environment, the carer pays attention to designing the physical environment in such a way as to facilitate a creative tension between home and adventure. One might offer the possibility of spatial experiences in which there is a transition between the familiar and unfamiliar in a way that is both nourishing and interesting. For example, a carer and the physically disabled person may expend some effort arranging a 'liminal' space near a window where the person can feel both at home with familiar things to hand, as well as the possibility of following the flights of birds as they venture to warmer climes. Well-being as a sense of abiding expanse is any place that stretches between home and adventure.

Temporal mobility: Future orientation

There is a well-being experience that emphasises a future orientation or future possibilities. When there is a sense of future orientation, a person may be tuned into the temporal possibilities of moving forwards into a future (either as a sense or literally) in ways that are valued or wanted. So, for instance, a sense of future orientation in a literal way may occur when one is able to identify and progress one's valued projects. Here, a person may be energised by life possibilities that call from the future and that motivate them in a way that constitutes a sense of purpose. This sense of meaningful purpose constitutes this kind of well-being because it can provide a quality of flow and continuity to the ongoing progression of one's life in time. Without this possibility one may feel 'stuck', as if frozen in time without meaningful invitations 'into the future'. A well-being future orientation may occur for example, as one looks forward to a celebration that is due to happen with others. Here, there is a well-being dimension in the anticipation of what is to be; a very human kind of joy. Well-being as future orientation does not need to be as special as this in order to act as a resource. One can imagine possibilities for achieving change in small ways that are welcome, anything that can provide a sense of new things happening and that constitute 'a breath of fresh air'. In relation to the implications for care, one can ask the question: what future orientation could be welcomed by this person, no matter how small? One example of a literal entry point into the possibility of facilitating future orientation could be where a carer considers, together with a person, those small changes that might 'unstick' a sense of deadening routine or situation. Well-being as a sense of temporal mobility is anything that offers an invitation into a welcoming future.

Temporal dwelling: Present centredness

There is a well-being experience that emphasises 'present centredness'.[5] When a person is absorbed in the present moment, they are tuned into a kind of temporal focus that offers 'at oneness', an intimacy, a sense of belonging or a deep connection with what is happening in the moment in ways that are valued or wanted. So for example, a sense of present centredness often occurs in marginal literal situations where one's attention 'is grabbed', such as in sports and other absorbing challenges. Here, people are 'in the zone'. An example in an everyday sense of temporal dwelling may be when one is enchanted by beautiful music or the taste of good food. In these and other situations, which may be very personal, one is 'brought home' to the very simple event of 'just being', and there is a completeness and satisfaction in this moment of temporal dwelling. In relation to the implications of this well-being emphasis for care, one can ask the question: what welcome present-centred experience can be facilitated and supported as a possible focus for experiential engagement? One example of offering a present focus to experience could be very simple such as the mere directing of a person's attention to something that is already there as a source of comfort, such as the gentle sound of rain on the roof or the rise and fall of breathing. Another example is where a sense of temporal dwelling is offered by helping the person to engage in activities of possible dwelling such as through painting, or through spending time in the garden. Well-being as a sense of present centredness is anything that offers absorption as a moment of welcome 'being here'.

Temporal dwelling-mobility: Renewal

There is a well-being experience that can hold a sense of temporal mobility and temporal dwelling together; an experience that unifies future orientation and present centredness at the same time. We call this experience 'renewal'. In 'renewal', a person is tuned into a temporal range that carries with it both the novelty of being called into the 'newness' of the future, as well the settledness of being absorbed in the present moment. There is simultaneously a welcome invitation from the future as well as a 'being here', present with whatever is happening. This is a 'rooted-flow', a sense of the present that strongly grounds the movement towards the future. The word 'renewal' indicates something of the freshness, aliveness and uniqueness of the present moment that has never before quite happened like this, as well as a sense of possibility and potential movement that leans towards a future that opens

5   We acknowledge that the Heidegger of *Being and Time* emphasises futurity (as we empha-sise in our section on temporal mobility). However, there are indications, following Mugerauer, that in Heidegger's later works on the topics of Dwelling and Gelassenheit, "to stand in the clearing" had a present-centred emphasis, even though none of the three ecstasies of time are ever alone or without one another.

up. Here, one is both intimately 'at one with the present moment', as well as energised by life's future possibilities; it is a dwelling that leans forward. So for example, a person may experience a feeling of being connected to their life's desires and their future possibilities through an activity, such as climbing towards the top of a mountain, as well as experiencing the 'nowness' of this 'complete moment' as it is unfolding. In relation to the implications of this well-being emphasis for care, one could ask the question: What possibilities for renewal can be offered in this person's situation? Here, one avenue of exploration concerns how meaningful ritual has characteristics that can mark the importance of the present moment, as well as signal the potential to move into a new phase or possibility as 'renewal'. So for example, in a situation of a person undergoing the kind of elective surgery that will involve the loss of a body part, a carer could facilitate something like 'a ritual' or some space and time by which the person is encouraged to honour that part of the body and its role in the past, and then move on to include some acknowledgement of what the new phase of life may open up. Well-being as a sense of renewal is any welcome 'joining' between the depth of the present and the openness of the future.

Intersubjective mobility: Mysterious interpersonal attraction

There is a well-being experience that emphasises 'mysterious interpersonal attraction'. When such attraction is present, a person is tuned into the inter-personal possibilities that offer movement (either metaphorically or literally) in ways that are valued or wanted. There is an 'eros' in which a person's 'otherness' is an attraction beyond any simple knowing. Indeed, the essence of this attractiveness is precisely in the mystery of otherness. This well-being possibility in the interpersonal realm constitutes an energised openness towards the other which can be called 'desire'. Such desire or attraction, when experi-enced as well-being, constitutes a kind of radiance and a 'leaning towards'. So for instance, a sense of mysterious interpersonal attraction may occur where one cannot quite name why it is that you wish to find out more about another person. The essence of this mysterious interpersonal attraction is not, however, in finding out or knowing that person, but in the sheer energy of the 'beyondness' of someone or something partially hidden in the unknown; this interpersonal unknown is always in a sense 'wild' (in the sense of undiscovered or exotic), an aliveness that energises an interest to reach towards the other, something that the spontaneous innocence of a baby's grasp understands. This gravitation towards the other is not only 'eros' but can also be 'agape': a respectful caring interest in the others difference and uniqueness. In relation to the implications for care, one can ask the question: what mysterious inter-personal attraction can be welcomed by this person as a source of interest in the world? One example of a literal entry point into the possibility of facilitating 'the spark' of the call from the mystery of otherness is where a carer surprises an animal lover who is withdrawing because of illness by bringing a new cat onto the scene. Well-being as a sense of mysterious interpersonal attraction is anything that offers an invitation into the mystery of being.

Intersubjective dwelling: Kinship and belonging

There is an interpersonal well-being experience that emphasises a sense of kinship and belonging. Here a person feels at home with another or others. This sense of familiar interpersonal connection constitutes relaxed situations of meeting in ways that can make us feel that we belong there. In such a metaphorical or literal situation of 'kinship' there is a sense of 'we' rather than 'I' and 'you'; an effortless being together with one another, a sense of familiar security and togetherness.

So for example, a sense of interpersonal kinship and belonging may occur literally where one has built up a long history with someone that one has come to love and know. However this sense of kinship and belonging can also occur in a more metaphorical way as when we meet a 'kindred spirit' with whom we feel immediately compatible on various levels such as personality, heritage, interest, and so on. In these situations of intersubjective dwelling there may be a kind of reconnecting with where we had left off previously, a long time ago, almost as if we share a kind of eternal presence with the other person. This may constitute the sense that not much time has passed once we are together again: there is an eternal return to dwelling in this interpersonal present. In relation to the implications of this well-being emphasis for care, one can ask the question: what forms of kinship and belonging can be facilitated and supported as a possible focus for experiential engagement? One example of a literal entry point into the possibility of facilitating a sense of kinship and belonging is where a carer, sensitive to the cultural background of a person, helps to connect that person with others from their shared background and to possible events, objects, music, and traditions from their heritage. Within this context, heritage can be healing in that it provides cultural homecomings and shelter. Alternatively a carer could facilitate a sense of kinship and belonging in a more metaphorical sense by engaging in shared stories in which the person remembers and where they can 'join with' ancestry and shared histories that give a sense of continuity, familiarity and belonging. Alternatively, some people may need interpersonal kinship experiences that move beyond the cultural level to include interests and affinities that are very specific and not necessarily related to cultural heritage. So for example 'clubs' and social networks have become much more important as the history of community life becomes more fragmented. Well-being as a sense of kinship and belonging occurs in any of the ways that one can find an 'at-homeness' with others.

Intersubjective dwelling-mobility: Mutual complementarity

There is an experience that can hold a sense of both intersubjective mobility and intersubjective dwelling together; an experience in which there is both the qualities of mysterious interpersonal attraction as well as kinship and belonging. We call this experience 'mutual complementarity'. In 'mutual complementarity', a person is tuned into the possibility of being with another or others in such a way that there is 'homelike-oneness' with the other, as well as an energetic separation or attractive mystery, 'calling' from the other. Here, there is a paradoxical quality of both familiarity and strangeness in which we are reciprocal but complementary to one another. The 'mutuality' is one of kinship and belonging, the complementarity is one of 'a giving' in which one is 'more' when together than when apart. So for example two or more people may have a sense of mutual complementarity when there is a partnership constituted by a shared equality, together with the ongoing learning that may come from each others difference. This is a creative tension of 'sameness' and difference'. The difference is given by a 'not knowing' in which the other appears as a mysterious depth that can be surprising and which brings something new to the relationship. At the same time a certain 'sameness' or familiar 'sharedness' is given by a familiarity based on a shared recognition of places where 'we meet' and that we have 'in common'. In this creative tension there is both the intimacy of feeling at home with the other, as well as a sense of the novelty that each brings to the other in a mutual and complementary way. Mutual complementarity as an intersubjective well-being experience is thus a journey of companionship that is both 'at home' and 'in adventure'. In relation to the implications of this well-being emphasis for care, one can ask the question: What forms of mutual complementarity can be facilitated and supported as a possible focus for experiential engagement? One example of a literal entry point into this possibility is where a carer encourages a couple who feel at home together but who are 'in a rut', to discover either things they do not yet know about each other or to pursue something new together. Alternatively a carer could facilitate a sense of mutual complementarity in a more metaphorical sense by helping a person engage with their cultural history in new ways that give new directions for that person's life, such as, an engagement with the cuisine of their culture that they had not previously known about. This opens up both an intersubjective reconnecting as well as a sense of new direction; something old and something new. Well-being as a sense of mutual complementarity can occur in any way that one finds the 'attractive unknown' in the ones that are close, and with whom we feel we belong.

Mood mobility: Excitement or desire

There is a well-being experience that emphasises the mood of excitement or desire. Here, well-being as a mood or felt attunement is emphasised, but specifically, as a mood which has the quality of movement and buoyancy. In everyday terms this mood may be characterised as one of excitement or welcome desire. So for example, there may be a sense of excitement when one is about to leave for a much longed-for holiday or special event. A sense of such excitement or desire in a metaphorical sense may occur when there is a feeling of possibility; a feeling that the world is inviting one into horizons that connect with the desires of one's heart. This energised feeling constitutes the mood of motivation, a kind of 'life force' or vitality that sustains the feeling that life is worth living. In relation to the implications of this 'well-being emphasis' for care, one can ask the question: what sense of excitement or desire in this person's situation can be offered? One example of offering an invitation to the mood of welcome excitement or desire may be in a situation where older people are living in a residential care setting. Here, such older people may be provided with opportunities to celebrate important events or seasons. In this example one is helping to focus attention on the possibility of a sense of celebration that brings with it a mood that has, in various ways, been available to us all as part of the heritage of being human. Well-being as a mooded sense of excitement is thus anything that motivates a felt connection to a person's meaningful life desires.

Mood dwelling: Peacefulness

There is a well-being experience that emphasises the mood of peacefulness. Here, well-being as a mood or felt attunement is emphasised, but specifically as a mood that has the qualities of stillness, settledness or reconciliation. In everyday terms this mood may be characterised as one of peace and welcome 'pause'. So for example, there may be a sense of peacefulness when one has fulfilled a task or responsibility that required some effort and commitment. We would like to note that the process of settling or 'coming to accept' things may be challenging, and that the direction of acceptance may be a journey that includes sadness, patience, and concern. A person can come to the mood of dwelling in multiple ways, but in the end, the mood of dwelling is one of peacefulness in spite of everything. A felt sense of peace may also be experienced in less literal situations through an attunement of mind, or through a more general comportment towards the world. Here, a person is able to accept 'what has been given' for what it is, and to experience the concomitant feeling of peacefulness that arises with such 'letting-be-ness'. Peace as a felt sense is thus the mood of dwelling or 'at-homeness'. In relation to the implications of this well-being emphasis for care, one can ask the question: what sense of peace or settledness is possible for this person? One literal example of offering an invitation to the mood of peace may be where a carer suggests, for example, that a person keeps 'a book of abundances' in which they note daily something that they can appreciate or accept 'just as it is'. A less literal example may be where a carer introduces practices that help focus a person's attention on the possibility of accepting things as they are, where it may be possible to do so. One can perhaps begin to encourage someone to do this by first noticing and appreciating simple changes in life such as the rhythms of day and night, and of the seasons, and the mood that this may bring. One could then move onto more complex mindful practices for life in which the possibility of peacefulness and 'letting be-ness' is progressively achieved as a general mood or comportment towards life's changes. Well-being as a mooded sense of peacefulness occurs whenever there is a felt acceptance of things, circumstances and changes.

Mood dwelling-mobility: Mirror-like multidimensional fullness

There is a well-being experience characterised by a highly complex mood that participates in both the energetic quality of enthusiasm and interest, as well as the settled quality of being at home with oneself and the world. We call this paradoxical mood 'mirror-like multidimensional fullness'. We have called this mood 'mirror-like' because it contains a settled openness that is large enough to reflect whatever is happening in a 'letting be' kind of way. At the same time we have called this mood 'multidimensional fullness' because it is a fullness of mood, which can be many things such as sadness, love and happiness. It can be many things because this mirror-like mood does not need to separate itself from whatever is happening right now. In not separating itself, the mood is one of 'union with', but a 'union with' the fluidity that is alive and unfolding, rather than a union with a finished circumstance. The paradoxical quality of the mood of 'mirror-like multidimensional fullness' is,
    metaphorically speaking, like that of being at both the centre and the periphery of a cyclone at the same time. There is a mood of both stillness and of being 'on the move' simultaneously. The mood is one of fullness in the sense that one feels complete and that nothing is missing; it is far from a sense of deficient emptiness. So for example, a person may experience a mood of mirror-like multidimensional fullness when they are 'drinking in' the novelty of new sights and sounds, and feeling complete 'there' in this moment. The paradoxical quality of this complex mood thus includes fullness and completeness, novelty and surprise, appreciation and serenity and so on. The Japanese Haiku tradition evokes something of this mood in stanzas such as:

how touching
to exist after the storm
chrysanthemum

(Basho 1692–94/ 2008)

In relation to the implications of this complex well-being mood for care, one could ask the question: what possibilities are there for such a complex mood that is one of 'giving oneself emotionally' to this moment, in both an enthusiastic and reconciled way. Sometimes this mood may occur spontaneously in a patient with a chronic illness after having 'gone through a lot'. Suddenly she feels something more than just acceptance and peace about her condition. She feels, without there being a reason, enthusiastic about sipping a simple cup of tea early in the morning. She is not enthusiastic in the sense of looking forward to anything, but in the sense that there is nothing more important to be or do, but just to fully 'give herself' to appreciating what is available now, even though there may be pain and uncertainty. This mood cannot be directly facilitated, and often comes in surprising and unexpected ways; it is the mood where hard-earned 'songs of experience' meet the child-like presence of 'songs of innocence'. It is not so much that professionals and carers can help make this happen, but that they can prevent this possibility from happening by not recognising or understanding the value of this mood, and therefore in such situations could mistakenly bring the person back prematurely to projections about the future, or back to a narrative definition of themselves. So, well-being as a sense of multidimensional fullness is characterised by the enthusiastic mood of 'giving oneself' to an experience without narrative implication, and because of, rather than in spite of, the limits of this timeless moment.

Identity mobility: 'I can'

There is a well-being experience that emphasises a sense of one's personal identity as 'I can'. When such an emphasis of personal identity is experienced, the person will experience themselves as being 'on the move' (either metaphorically or literally) in ways that are valued or wanted. Relating to their sense of personal identity, there is a sense of 'being able to', a degree of confident personal competence in which one feels able to move into the kind of future and its expanding horizons that are consistent with a knowledge of one's personal possibilities and self-belief. This sense of 'I can' can range from being very simple and literal to very complex and metaphorical. So, for example, this self-sense of 'being on the move' can be as simple as a toddler developing the self-belief that they can consistently walk to the corner. At a more complex and metaphorical level, this sense of 'I can' may occur when one has been able to develop a tacit sense of optimism that dreams can be realistically achieved on the basis of one's hard work and personal capacities. At its most existential level, there may be a very general sense that there is always 'a more' to one's identity, and a feeling that one's personal capacities lie in possible potentials that have not yet been named or realised. There is thus a very close relationship between 'I can' identity-mobility and a sense of personal agency. This well-being possibility in the realm of identity constitutes an energised openness about the possibilities of the self. In relation to the implications of this well-being emphasis for care, one could ask the question: what possibilities for self-efficacy are there in this person's life that are meaningful to the person and that can be offered and supported as either a literal reality or as a focus for possible experiential engagement? One example of facilitating a greater sense of self-efficacy may be with a person who has lost their confidence in being able to engage in past activities because of an illness. Here they can be encouraged to set small relevant goals, and over time, experience a gradual build-up of 'I can' successes. This 'I can' mobility-identity then becomes somewhat restored, and can constitute a source of well-being. An example that is less literal is where a more general sense of self-potential is facilitated. Here, a psychotherapy patient who had been overly identified with personal historical experiences of failure, may rediscover aspects of themselves, or previously unknown aspects of themselves that had been obscured by their self-definition of failure. This is usually done psychotherapeutically in a non-linear way where, instead of focusing on the problem, one helps the person to explore things about themselves and their potential that they may have forgotten. There are many ways in which this can be facilitated, for example, through art, writing, and through pursuing dormant passions. Well-being as a sense of 'I can' is thus any experience where one's personal identity is felt to be capable of 'being able to' and of being able to achieve what one values.

Identity dwelling: 'I am'

There is a well-being experience that is in touch with one's sense of personal identity as 'I am' in its most general sense. When such an emphasis of personal identity is in focus, a person may experience themselves as someone who is simply supported by histories and contexts that are continuous with one's sense of self, and which does not need to be excessively questioned or 'at stake'. This is not an 'I am' as if it were an objectified definition of oneself; rather it is an 'I am' that, at its depth, feels connected to a sense of being which is given to us in its most foundational sense. When one is tuned into this sense of identity, there is a sense of 'being there' before all the specific layers of self-definition that have been built up are brought into play. So, this sense of 'I am' is not 'I am this or that'; it really is just the feeling of 'being' very generally, or present, as 'someone who belongs here right now', and who is able to take 'nourishment' and some security from this sense of ontological identity. At its depth one can call it an 'ontological security': that one's identity (in a very general way) is supported by 'merely being' rather than 'having to be' something or someone. The well-being focus of the 'identity dwelling' emphasis of 'I am' is experienced as a familiar continuity, a sense of effortless connectedness, a certain peacefulness or lack of dilemma of who and what I am: a kind of being at home with one's self. In relation to the implications of this well-being emphasis for care, one can ask the question: what effortless or peaceful sense of 'I am' is possible for this person? One literal example of facilitating a greater sense of 'I am' that has an 'identity dwelling' quality, may be where one helps a disabled person connect with identity resources to which they feel continuous with, and belong to, beyond the particularity of 'I am disabled'. In this example a practitioner may facilitate the possibility of an experiential engagement in which the person recognises their continuity with cultural, geographical or historical connections with which they may identify such as a place, or a sense of belonging with 'my people'. A more existential example of deep 'identity dwelling' may be where a person who has been recently diagnosed with a terminal illness spontaneously realises, within the midst of their anguish, an inexplicable feeling that 'I am still here, and much more than my illness', and that 'my sense of being here' is vast and indefinable. At this existential level, such experiences cannot be predicted or determined, and seem to involve a kind of 'breakthrough' to a sense of self as 'simply being'. Such an ontological sense of the foundation of personal identity is a well-being resource in which a certain timeless dimension of one's depths relieves the narratives of our lives. Well-being as a sense of 'I am' is thus an experience where our sense of personal identity is felt to be connected to resources and contexts far beyond oneself, but which nevertheless, are continuous with what is most deeply one's own.

Identity dwelling-mobility: Layered continuity

There is a well-being experience that can hold a sense of identity-mobility and identity-dwelling at the same time; an experience that unifies 'I can' with 'I am'. We call this experience 'layered continuity'. In 'layered continuity' a person may experience their own identity, not in any particular thing like way, but as a sense of continuity with different layers of 'I can', as well as a continuity with the general sense of simply being here before all the specific layers of self-definition are brought to the fore. In this rare and paradoxical experience, both one's specific sense of identity, as well as one's strong sense of 'just being' in a foundational sense, are both in the foreground. Here, one's sense of identity is inclusive of a sense of all the historical details and connections that make up the 'I can', as well as the sense of ontological security of 'I am'. This sense of inclusion of both these identity resources is experienced as a layered continuity in which one is empowered by both the multiple resources of one's uniqueness as well as that level of identity that opens out to one's most anonymous and transpersonal ground. This layered continuity is thus continuous with both personal and transpersonal layers of self. Jung indicated this ambiguous experience of both the unity and multiplicity to one's identity when he said:

> . . . I am all these things at once and cannot hold up the sum . . . and it seems to me that I have been carried along. I exist on the foundation of something I do not know. In spite of all uncertainties I feel a solidity underlying existence and a continuity in my mode of being.
>
> (Jung, 1961/1995, p. 392)

The well-being experience in layered continuity lies in its inclusive qualities of 'I am all this and more'. So for example, a person may have a feeling of the 'layered continuity' of who they are in unguarded moments when the need to assert or protect any sense of self-definition is in abeyance; self-definition is not at stake and a sense of oneself as 'layers' that spontaneously shine through without the need to 'be achieved' is supportively experienced.

In relation to the implications of this well-being emphasis for care, one could ask the question: what possibilities are there for experiencing such a complex identity within this person's life situation? Again, such experiences cannot be predicted or determined, and seem to involve a kind of 'break-through' to an ambiguous sense of self as 'layered continuity'. An example of experiencing layered continuity may be in a person who has been through much effortful and self-conscious treatment regimes. After a long period in which she was struggling with her sense of self as 'a patient' trying to take 'full responsibility' for her recovery, she spontaneously realised, that there was not much more that she could do. Something deep within her relaxed; a letting go of the 'responsible one' and a 'letting in' of the deep need to simply be cared for. Suddenly in this moment, a sense of her layered continuity was restored; she felt unconcerned about any definition of herself that she had been upholding, and felt the well-being experience of 'I already am and I already can, even though I do not know who that is in specific terms – I am many layers'. Well-being as a sense of layered continuity is any experience where one's personal identity is felt to be both already achieved in its essence, as well as felt as a sense of self that is 'able to' in a general sense.

Embodied mobility: Vitality

There is a well-being experience that emphasises a sense of bodily 'vitality'. When there is such a sense of vitality a person may be tuned into an embodied energy that carries with it a quality of movement in ways that are valued or wanted. So for example a sense of embodied mobility may occur in a literal way, actualising the power of one's own body to move in various ways and towards different desired outcomes. This is a literal 'bodying forth'. Therefore, one important source of the kind of well-being that is given to bodily existence is an active power to move in, and with, one's world and others. At a more existential level, a sense of vitality can refer to energised bodily feeling that can occur without literal physical movement, such as in imagination, eroticism or any other generalised desire where one feels the energy of this motivation as a palpable bodily experience; it is an incarnate sense of vitality. This sense of vitality constitutes a kind of well-being because it essentially provides life-forward and life-positive qualities of 'being an actor' or 'agent' in the world; of extending one's power freely, a 'life force' in the world through bodily sensation and capacity. Without this possibility one may feel depleted and lacking in bodily energy and functional capacity. In relation to the impli-cations of this well-being emphasis for care contexts one could ask the question: what possibilities for bodily vitality can be offered and supported to this person as either a literal reality or as a focus for possible experiential engagement? A literal example of the possibility of restoring a sense of vitality may be where a physiotherapist works with a person to maximise a dysfunctional limb so that literal movement is enhanced. Further literal examples of restoring a sense of vitality refer to all the ways in which vitality can be restored on a biomedical level by attending to the physiological basis of depletion, ill health or lack of function. An example of facilitating a sense of vitality in a more metaphorical or existential way may occur in the case of a person who is experiencing an embodied listlessness and lethargy. Here, a carer may understand that this bodily listlessness and lethargy is not disconnected from the person's felt sense of 'how' or 'where' their life is going, where they feel blocked, and where there may be possibilities for moving forward.

With such an understanding, the carer may help the person to first see a link between their bodily sense of lethargy and the blocked life projects that are announced. Secondly, the carer may help the person to then focus their energies on meaningful possibilities that are relevant to them. If this is successful, the sense of existential movement achieved will concurrently constitute the more bodily felt level of 'movement' that we are calling vitality. Well-being as a sense of vitality thus occurs as the bodily sense of refreshed possibilities in literal and metaphorical ways.

Embodied dwelling: Comfort

There is a well-being experience that is in touch with one's sense of 'comfort' as a bodily experience. When such a sense of bodily comfort is felt, a person may literally experience their body as warm, full, relaxed, still, satiated, rooted. Here one feels a welcome simple sense of 'being at home' in one's body, simply feeling the support or nourishment of the reliable rhythms of one's natural bodily functions, as in the gentle rise and fall of the breath or the relaxation of the body at rest. In bodily comfort there is a certain unforced sense of familiarity and intimacy with the internal natural and organic rhythms announced by the body. There are also silent and unseen rhythms that we take for granted but which support the palpable sense of comfort. Such natural comfort is, in a sense unthought or pre-reflective. The comfortable body is simply there in its reliable givenness. Here, one is unpreoccupied with the body. The body does not announce itself as a dilemma'; it 'just is' and is in 'letting be' mode. We know comfort through a kind of trust rather than through a purposeful search. At its depths such bodily comfort is connected to natural rhythms beyond oneself such as the rhythms of day and night, warmth and coolness, and other fleshly contexts that are familiar to a body that feels comfortable in its context. We can also think of the comfort of bodily dwelling in a more metaphorical way as in Mary Oliver's (2004) expression your '*soft animal body*', a body 'curled up' or 'folded in' with sources of nourishment and support, sustaining a bodily sense of well-being. Metaphorically we could say that the body knows that it comes from primordial darkness, intimate with rhythms within rhythms, lapping on this fleshly shore. Bodily comfort as well-being is something the body deeply knows as a tacit, self-evident foundation to healthy being. Comfort constitutes a kind of well-being because it essentially provides an embodied dwelling in which there are qualities of 'non-purposeful natural presence' as a foundation for being there. Such comfort is a bodily 'gravitas' that makes possible an embodied openness to the world. Without comfort as a well-being possibility, one may feel a sense of *dis*-ease, a preoccupation with the palpable bodily sense that 'something is wrong'. In relation to the implications of this well-being emphasis for care, one can ask the question: what possibilities for bodily comfort are available to this person at either a literal or existential level? A literal example of the possibility of restoring a sense of comfort will be familiar to many readers. Here for example, a carer may aim to bring comfort to a paralysed person through being sensitive to the need for a change of position, and to facilitate a welcome refreshment through bathing, clean linen, a warm drink, and with attention to minimising noise and bright light. Again, there are also many literal ways in which comfort can be facilitated by a medical means. A more existential example of promoting a sense of comfort may occur in the case of an immigrant who is experiencing bodily restlessness and insomnia. Here, a professional may understand this restlessness and insomnia in a way that is not disconnected from the person's felt sense of 'trying to find a way back home', where home in a literal sense is no longer available. With such an understanding, the professional may help the person to find bodily reminders of feeling at home, perhaps through familiar foods or other possible ways that connect the person to the bodily feeling of comfort of what home is like for them. If this is successful to some degree, the sense of existential settling that is achieved may also constitute the more bodily level of comfort that provides enough security to perhaps 'settle' and sleep. Well-being as a sense of comfort thus occurs as the bodily sense of 'feeling at home' and settling in literal and metaphorical ways.

Embodied dwelling-mobility: Grounded vibrancy

There is a well-being experience that can hold a sense of embodied mobility and embodied dwelling at the same time, an experience that unifies vitality with comfort. We call this experience 'grounded vibrancy'. In grounded vibrancy a person's bodily existence is felt as an intertwining of gentle energised flow, unified with a bodily sense of feeling deeply at home and settled. In this complex experience, there may be a bodily sense of both 'being' and 'becoming' at the same time; a sense of fullness that solidly anchors the body and with it, a 'humming' vibrancy that is attracted to unfinished horizons. This paradoxical quality of grounded vibrancy contains both a sense of the freshness of renewal and great possibility, as well as a sense of the deep continuity that belongs to feeling 'at one with' oneself and the world. This bodily well-being experience can be expressed more poetically as a 'well-spring, a bubbling brook at its source, from the ground'. The bodily feeling where being and becoming 'are humming' can constitute a welcome and effortless bodily tension or oscillation between the body's 'quest' (the attraction to unfinished horizons) and satiation (the comfort of bodily fulfilment). The body's 'quest' is given by a certain kind of vitality that is the essence of the feeling of 'being attracted'. At the same time a bodily sense of comfort is experienced at a deeper level in the background. This background bodily sense of completeness and tranquillity holds and empowers a bodily vibrancy that is 'ticking over' with potential, and a readiness to live forward. In relation to the implications of this well-being emphasis for care, one could ask the question: what possibilities are there that would allow a person to experience grounded vibrancy? Because of the complexity of this experience, its circumstance cannot be determined or predicted: situations that facilitate either comfort or vitality can make way for it. But there is something 'extra' to the comfort or vitality. So, for example, we were told a story by one of our friends about a man with dementia. He is outside with his carer on a hot day, and sees an ice-cream van. He does not know what to call it, but points, and his carer buys him one. He tastes and his eyes light up. He looks for words but can't find them, so exclaims: "This is a good one!!" Here, there is a deep bodily satisfaction and recognition as well as an enthusiasm that links the body's 'satiation' to the vibrant world of a 'hot-summer's-day-full-of -ice-cream-potential'. Well-being as a sense of grounded vibrancy is any bodily experience where variations of rest and comfort are intertwined with variations of alertness and vitality,

Conclusion

Although we have given examples of specific possible ways that each of the well-being emphases can be facilitated within a caring context, such experiential possibilities should not be understood in a deterministic way as if certain conditions will inevitably lead to certain well-being experiences. Within the human realm, experiential well-being possibilities can happen unpredictably in spontaneous and unexpected ways. The conditions for well-being such as economic, political, social, health -related, and institutional, may provide either a support or an obstruction to well-being, but these conditions are not always sufficient or necessary for the experience of well-being to occur. This existential view of well-being is thus consistent with a resource-oriented approach in which the possibilities for well-being experiences can be revealed or focused upon from the perspective of its widest literal and deepest existential contexts. By considering the multidimensional facets of well-being as articulated in this framework, we may widen and complexify the range of possible resources that are available for the alleviation of suffering. Here, suffering is much more complex than illness, and well-being is much more complex than health. In our view it is this multidimensional complexity that defines the deepest and broadest lifeworld directions for caring.

We would also like to say something about the deepest possibility of well-being as a developmental calling. There is obviously a relationship between 'existence' and 'caring', but well-being as an existential call far exceeds the vocation of caring. The existential theory of dwelling-mobility also has implications for a broader quest towards well-being as an existential task. For example, a further development of the theory could focus on an articulation of the deepest possibilities of well-being as 'an existential pull' in peoples' lives. Future elaboration of the theory would then focus on the developmental processes by which human attention can be widened in such a way as to sustain multiple intertwined dimensions of well-being as an increasingly available conscious resource at the foundation of experiential life.

Having acknowledged the existential developmental task that is given by the call of well-being, we would like finally to come back to the importance of our theory of well-being for the project of caring. In the midst of suffering, a felt experience of well-being is particularly important to people as an inner resource when they are facing health-related challenges. Carers can then become much more attuned to the importance and value of this felt experience for the person. The wider 'vocabulary' for well-being experiences that are offered here, may contribute to an emerging cultural discourse that wishes to put well-being as a value more centrally at the forefront of public life.

7 Kinds of suffering
Caring for vulnerability

In this chapter, following a similar logic to the preceding chapter concerning the different kinds and levels of well-being, we offer an existential theory of suffering and a framework that delineates eighteen kinds of suffering. There are two reasons why we wish to complement a focus on well-being with a focus on suffering: Firstly, we see a continuum of well-being and suffering, although not a linear continuum in which one excludes the other; well-being and suffering are always in relation to one another. Secondly, various discourses have either overemphasised well-being and obscured the significance of suffering, or overemphasised suffering and obscured the well-being possibilities. We believe that a humanly sensitive care that matters requires a view and understanding of both: a focus on well-being provides a direction for care; and a focus on, and understanding of, suffering, provides a human capacity for care. This dual focus is consistent with the view of the person articulated in Chapter 3 where we argued that it is important to meet people in both their vulnerabilities as well as their possible freedoms: suffering announces vulnerability, and well-being announces freedom.

Our existential theory of suffering and the framework that delineates eighteen kinds of suffering is also derived from Heidegger's concern with 'homecoming', as well as the fundamental constituents of human experience that we employed in our theory of well-being. We were sensitised by his inclusive approach of holding both 'homelessness' and 'homecoming' in relation to one another. His descriptions of 'homelessness' provide the possibilities of a deep existential understanding of human vulnerability and suffering (for example, finitude). His later writings provide, although often indirectly, some deep existential understandings of the possibility of well-being (releasement). His later optimism about 'letting-be-ness' did not eradicate a keen tragic sensibility, and we think that he was interesting in the way that he embraced both the tragic and the transcendental or emancipatory dimensions of life. We now describe our framework for delineating different kinds and levels of suffering.

As in our previous chapter, on the left hand side of Table 7.1 we name a number of experiential domains within which suffering can be emphasised (spatiality, temporality, intersubjectivity, etc.). Along the horizontal rows the two emphases of suffering (dwelling and mobility) are delineated together

Table 7.1 A framework for delineating different kinds and levels of suffering

	MOBILITY	DWELLING	DWELLING-MOBILITY
SPATIALITY	Imprisoned	Exiled	Roomless
TEMPORALITY	Blocked future	Elusive present	No respite
INTER-SUBJECTIVITY	Aversion	Alienated isolation	Persecution
MOOD	Depression	Agitation	Restless gloom
IDENTITY	I am unable	I am an object or 'thing'	I am fragmented
EMBODIMENT	Stasis and exhaustion	Bodily discomfort and pain	Painful closing down

with a third possibility when intertwined or unified (dwelling-mobility). The terms 'dwelling' and 'mobility' are used in the same way as in our well-being theory and we refer readers to those definitions and meanings. Again, as in the previous chapter, by considering the relative interaction of these two dimensions (experiential domains and suffering possibilities), one can derive a number of kinds of suffering that are afforded to human existence.

Mobility suffering in the spatial dimension: Imprisoned

There is a suffering experience that emphasises a sense of spatial imprisonment. A person may feel hemmed in, unable to move, trapped, with no room or any horizon that can give respite. When a person experiences such a sense of 'contracted horizon' or lack of room to move, there is a claustrophobic feeling, which at its extreme may constitute either the panic of wanting to get out, or the despair of being cramped or locked in.

So for example, when a person gives over their body for critical care, with all the restrictive technology that this necessarily requires such as intravenous lines and monitoring equipment, their world shrinks to the immediate bed space around them and their spatial horizons are emptied of choice or possibility.

Or imagine a more metaphorical example of the sense of needing more or different space. For example, a relationship can be claustrophobic or oppressive and a person may need to go for a long walk in the fresh air to remind them of the possibility of a more 'open free space'.

A carer or practitioner's sensitivity to the meaning of this kind of spatial suffering can equip him or her to meet the person 'there', and to be sensitive to the need for some kind of 'freedom in space' whether literally or meta-phorically. Even if greater spatial mobility is not possible, such sensitivity to the meaning of this dimension may help to reduce the person's sense of imprisonment. Suffering as a sense of imprisonment is anything that constrains a wished for change of movement or spatial horizons.

Dwelling suffering in the spatial dimension: Exiled

There is a suffering experience that emphasises a sense of spatial exile. A person may feel cast out into an inhospitable place, wrenched from a familiar space, banished to an alien place with limited opportunity for relief or breathing space. When a person experiences such a sense of inhospitable constraint, there may be a sense of 'being thrown' into a noxious place with no way back. They may feel separated which, at its extreme, may constitute a feeling of estrangement and alienation, and a sense of being far from home with a painful longing for a return to a place where we belong.

So for example, some people may not find it difficult to fall asleep in a hospital room with overhead artificial lighting. However, for another person the environment may feel intensely 'un-homelike' and impersonal, making it impossible to settle. Here, whatever suffering the person may be experiencing may be compounded by this sense of spatial exile and there may be an intense feeling of longing for familiar sights, sounds and rhythms, and a deep pang for home. Here the practitioner may not understand what appear to be small irritations of the patient, for example, wanting to block out the light in order to constitute 'a kind of cave'.

Or imagine a more metaphorical example of someone who has a wanderlust and spends much of her life moving from place to place. She can't quite articulate the kind of place that she is looking for, but feels a restlessness and a certain sense of painful exile. There is a spatiality to the sense of 'something missing' in that it is searched for 'out there', but the characteristic of this particular kind of spatial exile is that it is nameless. It is hard to know what would constitute spatial homecoming for this person.

A practitioner who is sensitive to the kind of suffering that is 'spatial exile' is more equipped to be sensitive to forms of caring that do not further exacerbate the sense of a person's exile. Such care can simply be based on the understanding of the importance of hospitality even if this is not literally possible. Suffering as a sense of exile is any place that feels unwelcome.

Dwelling-mobility suffering in the spatial dimension: Roomless

There is a roomless hell in which the spatial qualities of both exile and imprisonment are intertwined. In such roomlessness one is not just longing for home but is so trapped in homelessness that there is the despair of 'little or no possibility'. This roomlessness is darker than the anxiety of entrapment or the longing of exile. Exile on its own without entrapment carries with it the intended possibility of home. Imprisonment on its own, without exile, carries with it the potential of a freedom that would be worthwhile, worth waiting or fighting for. But in roomlessness there is no future place 'worth looking for' and one is imprisoned there. This constitutes a despair that is deeper than either the anxiety of entrapment on its own, or the experience of longing that comes with 'exile' on its own: there is nowhere to return to. One can imagine extreme literal possibilities of roomlessness such as being taken away to places that have no way back, and such situations would require complex literal solutions such as in 'The Jungle Book', where there is no ready-made home to come back to. However, roomlessness as a metaphorical or existential condition may be much more common. Suffering as a sense of roomlessness refers to all the spatial ways that one can be imprisoned with no sense of meaningful place beyond that to aspire to, or to return to.

Mobility suffering in the temporal dimension: Blocked future

There is a suffering that emphasises a sense of temporal stagnation. A person may feel 'stuck' in the deadening sense that there is no way to move forward in time. They may feel blocked or cut off from any sense of the future.

When a person experiences such lack of temporal mobility there is very little from the future that invites them. A sense of meaningful purpose recedes, and the present becomes an oppressive repetition. The future has closed down. At its extreme this feeling may constitute a sense of life being stopped in its tracks and a person may feel frozen in time.

So for example, imagine receiving some unexpected bad news. Time can stand still. In 'the shock of it', the future may suddenly no longer make much sense in terms of one's existing motivations and meaningful personal projects. This can be a phase in a natural rhythm, but for various reasons, one can become stuck here and experience the ghost-like suffering of being in 'no man's land' or 'limbo'. What does it take for the future to become inviting once again?

A carer who is sensitive to the meaning of this kind of temporal suffering is appreciative of the importance of 'a sense of journey' for people. Such a carer is always seeking opportunities by which they can at least invite a person into 'small steps forward' from where a future can meaningfully call. Suffering as a sense of blocked future refers to any times in one's life where the possibilities for meaningfully moving forward recede or even stand still; a living in the doldrums with no wind in the sails.

Dwelling suffering in the temporal dimension: Elusive present

There is a suffering that emphasises a sense of temporal unsettledness. Here, for various reasons, a person may feel unable to 'stand still' either because the present moment is unpleasant or because the 'pull' of the past or the future has excessive obscuring power. One is unable to simply 'be present' then; there is either an excessive 'running towards' or a 'running away'.

There are many variations of this kind of temporal suffering, particularly in these times when 'tick tock time' has become persecutory. But all these variations result in the core existential dilemma of 'life passing oneself by', stripping the present of its vividness, almost as if there was no good time to be there. Sometimes one can force oneself to inhabit the present moment by strong measures such as extreme sports or other absorbing pursuits. This reminds one of the kind of 'well-being' made possible when one is able to unambivalently inhabit the present moment.

An example of the suffering given by the 'elusiveness of the present' is where a person is so desperately fixed on a future dream that they are seldom able to relax and appreciate what is happening around them. In quieter moments they feel an anxious restlessness and need to quickly occupy themselves with some activity that distracts them from the feeling that this moment is never good enough. Here the future is too demanding and wields its manic power. Alternatively the possibility of welcoming the present may be excessively obscured by the traumatising power of the past. Here, a person may be constantly looking backwards to 'ghosts and fears' that possess the present. There is an anxious dread and the present can only be inhabited by a guarded vigilance. All of us can recognise various degrees of such everyday suffering but one can imagine levels of such suffering in which a lack of temporal dwelling visits and grips.

A carer or practitioner who is sensitive to the meaning of this kind of temporal suffering will look for opportunities in which they can help people to slow down and perhaps begin to feel the kind of permission required to immerse themselves in small and simple moments. Suffering as a sense of the 'elusive present' refers to any happening that cannot be inhabited and welcomed, and constitutes a range of suffering experience, from numbness to restlessness to ambivalence to extreme anguish.

Dwelling-mobility suffering in the temporal dimension: 'No respite'

There is a hell of 'no respite' in which the temporal qualities of both a blocked future and an elusive present are intertwined. There are a number of variations of this temporal form of suffering but in its most intense forms, the present is intolerable and the future is repellent. In such an 'eternity of suffering' neither the future nor the present provide possibilities of respite. Such a condition of no respite is different from a blocked future on its own, whereby one may still take refuge in one's present situation, even though one cannot see where this is going. It is also different from an elusive present where although one is unable to settle in one's present circumstances, a hoped-for future may still be meaningful to the person as a possibility. In 'no respite' one is truly between a rock and a hard place in which one is lost in a limbo that is relentless. This constitutes an anguish and a despair that is deeper than either the oppression of a blocked future on its own, or the restlessness or running away from a present that is unpalatable. In milder variations of 'no respite' there is a 'restless aimlessness', and in more intense variations, the relentlessness of suffering speaks only of repetition; no way out.

A carer who is bearing witness to or being with someone who is 'in a time of no respite' can err in two ways: on the one hand the carer may need to deny that no respite exists as an existential or literal condition. In such a case the patient can feel the additional suffering of an abandonment in which she has to bear the lonely burden of the depth and meaning of this suffering not being acknowledged by another. On the other hand, in the case of a carer who is able to fully acknowledge the reality of the despair and anguish of 'no respite' for the patient, the carer may prematurely collude with the hopelessness in the suffering and be constrained to seeking simplistic literal ways out. To limit ourselves to a world that assumes to know only literal solutions, either good or bad, is to deny existential possibilities far beyond simplistic models of causality. Suffering as a sense of 'no respite' refers to different variations of the times of one's life that feel unliveable, with no way forward.

Mobility suffering in the intersubjective dimension: Aversion

There is a suffering that emphasises an aversion towards being with another or others. The energy of this interpersonal aversion polarises the 'Me' from the 'You', and I either become the one who feels the aversion, or the one who is the victim of the aversion towards me. This is the realm of interpersonal conflict and its shades. In its mildest forms there is merely a lack of energetic interest in another or others; an absence of attraction, a boredom, a looking for someone else. When a person experiences such a lack of *Eros* in its broadest sense, life may lose its interpersonal spark, the potential mobility of interpersonal attraction and the fulfilments it brings. When the energy of *Eros* is not just absent but turns into aversion, there may then be an active desire of wanting to move away from another or others, and if the desired privacy or distance is not achieved, the person is then trapped in the suffering of interpersonal toxicity. Alternatively, when you are not interested or attracted to me, I feel invisible, or in a more extreme version, feel 'ugly' or full of shame. Thus the more extreme polarised forms of this kind of interpersonal suffering result in either a humiliation or a disgust.

Within the context of health and social care there is a therapeutic eros that is different from a sexual eros (Boss, 1963). Here, one dimension of care is to energetically care for another's possibilities, almost as if one is standing on behalf of their flourishing. This 'eros', when absent, can make a patient feel merely like a number or a statistic. But more than this, if a carer's orientation turns into interpersonal aversion, a patient can feel the kind of humiliation that can make them at best want to hide, and at worst, to wish to die. This is an example of being the victim of interpersonal disinterest or aversion. And then, from the other side there is also the example of a patient losing their own interpersonal spark because of illness. For example, imagine a person who used to dance a lot, and through illness, could no longer be attracted to the joys of interpersonal invitation in this way. When he could no longer dance, a world of meaningful intersubjective mobility had fallen away and there was little invitation at the level he had. Illness for him is not then adequately described by the lack of quantitative mobility. A carer who is sensitive to this kind of suffering in which a certain vital connection with others has become impossible because of illness, will understand something of his loss: a whole pathway to others has receded and he is faced with the prospect of trying to fill this hole. One needs to understand what a dance is to understand this kind of suffering. In essence, interpersonal disinterest or aversion is thus a form of suffering in which the attractive dimensions of interpersonal life have gone far away or have even become a source of disgust or humiliation.

Dwelling suffering in the intersubjective dimension: Alienated isolation

There is an interpersonal suffering that emphasises the experience of alienation and isolation from others. Here, one's sense of interpersonal belonging and kinship is ruptured in various ways and to various degrees. One may be cast out and exiled, forced to roam far away from the interpersonal warmth of 'one's people'. Or one may feel a stranger in a room full of others. Loneliness can be literal, but it can also be existential. So for example, a person may feel uninvited or even excluded from interpersonal connection. There may be a feeling of being cut off from others, 'wronged' or even cast out from meaningful engagement. One is a 'foreigner' or out- sider. At its extreme, a person may feel isolated and may sense an inhos- pitable lack of belonging. When a person experiences such a lack of kinship there is no invitation to join in, and suffering may be experienced as a deep loneliness, a longing for familiar interpersonal connection, or even the pain of feeling like an unwanted outsider or pariah. There are many variations of this kind of intersubjective suffering but all are characterised by a core existential dilemma of having no interpersonal home or sense of belonging with others. In literal or metaphorical ways one is a foreigner, an exile, an outcast, a stranger.

Let us take a subtle but everyday example. Those of us who are 'health and social care professionals' may take for granted the professional inter-personal world to which we belong. Being part of this professional world may give us a sense of familiarity, the 'we world' where we are part of an 'in-group'. We thus may become easily desensitised to the experiences of alienation and lack of belonging that a patient may experience when entering this milieu. But even more than this, we may take a subtle satisfaction in emphasising the conditions for interpersonal acceptance. It needs quite a lot of personal and professional reflexivity to step back from perpetrating this kind of 'inhospitality'. But patients are acutely sensitive at such times in their life to this vulnerability. The suffering of alienated isolation occurs whenever there is a painful rupture to interpersonal belonging, whether literally or existentially.

Dwelling-mobility suffering in the intersubjective dimension: Persecution

There is a persecuted hell where aversion to others and alienated isolation are intertwined. There are many variations of this interpersonal form of suffering, but in its most extreme forms, one may feel at great threat from others with no way out. Here, others have become the source of one's pain and threat. One may feel oneself as an outsider whose very existence is not wanted. In some variations one feels victimised. This condition of persecuted interpersonal suffering, whether literal or existential, is deeper than aversion on its own or lonely isolation on its own. Aversion on its own carries with it a background interpersonal world in which there is still the possibility of an attractiveness or a benign other calling one out from the aversion or a buffering of oneself against the aversion. Alternatively there is the possibility of alienated isolation on its own without aversion. Here, one still wants to come home to the familiarity of interpersonal warmth that seems possible. However, in persecution, trust is lost; aversion and alienated isolation lock each other in. In this 'locked in' form of interpersonal hell a person is ensnared in a noxious interpersonal context. Not only is there a painful rupture of interpersonal belonging but there is the threat of destruction by others. Such persecution carries with it the possibility of both despair and terror. The despair is constituted by a lack of hope of being relieved from the condition of lonely isolation; the terror is constituted by the relentless threat of what others have become in the absence of a 'redeeming light'.

One can imagine extreme literal possibilities of persecution, banishment and dispossession. But in everyday terms, let us imagine a person who is about to be admitted to hospital. She was incarcerated during the Second World War. The institutional place that she had been in was not just a dwelling of non-belonging but a dwelling of great threat. Today, any suggestion of a hospital environment then ignites a world of institutions that are not just unhomely, but also aversive; these places become persecutory. When admitted to hospital she becomes much worse and no one appears to know why. A carer who is sensitive to this kind of interpersonal suffering can appreciate how being trapped in a context of interpersonal persecution can contribute to deterioration into deep despair and even terror. An understanding of the complexity of this intertwined form of interpersonal suffering may help carers develop the kind of patience and tolerance in which they realise that the re-establishment of the possibility of trust cannot be rushed, and to begin to think about the small steps of support that may still be meaningful to the person. In essence, suffering as persecution refers to all the ways that one can become subject to the dual injury of both threat and banishment.

Mobility suffering in mood: Depression

There is a form of suffering that emphasises a 'closed in' mood of limited or dark horizons. The mood of depression is characterised by a lack of energy and motivation, an uninviting future, a kind of dullness, a pessimistic outlook, a painful sense of not being able to carry on. There are many variations and nuances to this mood of depression, but all kinds and levels are constituted by a felt inability to move forward; one feels weighed down and helplessly stuck there. Implicit in its variations there may be a sense of unworthiness, a feeling of guilt, hopelessness, despair, or even a desire to die. There may be different kinds and levels of self hate and anger. As a deficit of 'mood mobility', depression is a powerful counterforce to the lightness and flexibility of experiential life-flow with its welcome vibrant colours. Depression is mostly dark or grey. There is little excitement and the call of eros becomes thwarted in different ways.

An understanding of all these different nuances of depression are particularly important in health care situations where this mood becomes intimately intertwined with a person's experience of illness. Imagine for example a person who has been experiencing chronic pain for a number of years. Carers who understand the complexity of pain and how the experience of pain intertwines with the mood of depression know that physical pain can induce many of the qualities of the mood of depression: a lack of energy, an uninviting future, a dullness, a sense of not being able to carry on. Such carers will be very attentive to ways in which they can address these nuances, both by medical means, such as medication and other interventions, as well as by lifeworld means such as by facilitating physical and motivational movement in both literal and metaphorical ways. Such care includes helping the person to accept limitations and what they have had to let go of, and to find or recover a renewed life project or possibility. The essence of suffering as a mood of depression refers to any of the felt qualities of gloom that comes with an unwilling loss of vital desire and the consequent diminution of motivation, energy and interest.

Dwelling suffering in mood: Agitation

There is a form of suffering that emphasises the mood of unsettled restlessness. This mood of agitation is characterised by a feeling of irritation, anxiety, disturbance, a sense that something is wrong. This agitated mood has a number of variations all of which involve a mild or intense feeling of wanting one's present circumstance to change, to be different or to stabilise. One may either feel like a leaf in the wind, hurried along, or like a gathering storm, forcefully pushing aside all in its midst. There is a feeling that one needs to fight against outside forces that are impinging, a feeling of relentless inter-ference from outside. Whichever nuance of agitation is emphasised, there is a felt quality of unpleasantness, a lack of harmony to the way one is met by things and circumstance, 'not right', 'too hot', 'too cold'. There is an unplea-sant 'lack of fit' between oneself and the world: either a wanting for what is elusive or an aversion to what presents itself. In such an agitated mood, anxiety is never far away, and announces the literal or existential situation of never feeling at home; a rupture to dwelling. As a deficit of 'mood dwelling' agitation is a powerful counterforce to simply settling into or dwelling with what is there, whether pleasant or unpleasant. So, the mood of agitation is often self-sustaining as it is a 'running away' that continues to need 'to run away', or a 'running after' that continues to need to run after. In agitation, there is a kind of excitability, but an unpleasant kind that only motivates the wish to escape, or the wish to grasp what eludes one.

As a carer in a health and social care context, it may become particularly important to recognise the energy of agitation and what it is trying to achieve. For example imagine a person who is struggling to accept their diagnosis. A carer may understand their agitation as a need to 'be in denial' for a while. The movement from this agitated defence to a dealing with the anxiety that may come up in 'dwelling' with the reality of the diagnosis, is a rhythmical process that needs to be respected. A carer would interact with the person in a way that provides sufficient time for the complexities of this mooded task: the back and forth rhythms between agitation and anxious dwelling. The essence of suffering as a mood of agitation refers to any of the felt qualities of unpleasant restlessness that comes with the need to defend oneself or run away from impinging, interfering or threatening forces.

Dwelling-mobility suffering in mood: Restless gloom

There is a hell of restless gloom where the moods of depression and agitation are intertwined. There are a number of variations of this mood of suffering, but in its most intense forms, one may feel a gloom that is intolerable; the intensity of this is such that it agitates us to find any way out. The fantasies of escape are extreme but are all characterised by a desire to end everything, if necessary, as there is an unconditionality about the global nature of this 'double whammy' of gloom and agitation. Everyday life may feel like a living nightmare and the relentless mood of this feels too overwhelming to endure. The emotional pain is such that there is a restless preoccupation for some kind of respite whether it be in sleep, numbness or death. The tortuous qualities of this mood however are such that one feels helpless to engineer respite, and one is left with an inconsolable gloom. This gloom is too big to fully feel and so one is trapped in a liminal space between being condemned to the feeling, and at the same time, being preoccupied with running away from it. This painful liminal mood of restless gloom is different from depression on its own, or agitation on its own. In depression on its own, one may give oneself to the simple energy of being dragged down, defeated, squashed, giving up, extinguished, flattened, lost. In agitation on its own, one does not stay still enough to be grabbed by the gloom; there is a strong impulse to be in another place, in another time, in another body, but the full mood of what one is running away from does not often break through to be fully felt. Alternatively, in the intertwining of restless gloom, one is truly between 'a rock and a hard place'. Here, nothing helps; the gloom relentlessly surrounds one, and even though one is agitatedly focused on distracting strategies, none are successful. In less intense variations of restless gloom there may be a sense of quiet desperation, a nervous helplessness, and an insatiable reaching after unreachable compensations.

It is not hard to imagine the marginality of this kind of suffering and the terrible dilemma of carrying an unrelenting and overwhelming dark mood that colours everything. Such a mood may feel as if it is deep inside oneself, and indeed feels as if it *is* oneself: it goes wherever one is. Restless gloom can be experienced by anyone in different situations and circumstances, and is not necessarily just connected with mental health issues. Let us take, for example, a person's cancer journey. Imagine the phase where it dawns on a person that the treatment is not working. The cancer feels deep inside, and they feel as if a bridge has been crossed where, in a sense, the cancer is taking over and possessing them, even 'becoming them'. There may be a mood of restless gloom. A carer who is able to understand this intertwined mood to some degree will not deny the gravity of it on the one hand. Here he offers meaningful existential company. But on the other hand, he offers something that may be missed by the depth of the gloom: that we can never know absolutely and that there is always change. It is in this caring for the 'not knowing' that the carer is able to then say 'let's go on a little bit'.

Mobility suffering in the identity dimension: 'I am unable'

There is an experience of suffering that emphasises a sense of one's personal identity as 'I lack ability'. When one is carrying this meaning of personal identity, the person may experience themselves as being 'useless' or 'failed' (either metaphorically or literally). Relating to one's sense of personal identity, there is a sense of 'not being able to', a degree of incompetence, a lack of confidence, self-belief, self-efficacy, a pessimism about one's self capacities, all leading to a felt sense that one will not be able to change anything in meaningful ways. One feels helpless, even despairing about one's abilities. At its depth, there is a contracted self-enclosure, and there may be a rigid identification with a conclusion about one's 'uselessness'. This may then become the filter or lens by which one's possibilities are negatively viewed. This sensed lack of personal ability can range from being very simple and literal to very complex and metaphorical. So, for example, this 'I am unable' can be as simple as lacking personal confidence to step onto an escalator. At a more complex level, this self perception that 'I lack ability' can become a pervasive sense of failure about the possibility of being able to do 'what it takes' to achieve aspirations that are valued. Existentially, there may be a very general sense that one is painfully lacking in certain capacities. This often occurs together with a fearful and potentially humiliating 'sinking feeling' that one will be 'found out' as incompetent. There is thus a very close relationship between the 'I am unable' identity mobility and a sense of a lack of personal agency. This suffering in the realm of identity lies in its energised feeling of personal uselessness, and when the pain of this escalates, it may develop into a self-destructive impulse, a fantasy of wanting to destroy oneself as the 'failed one': 'if I am unable, I should not be'. At this extreme level the emotional pain may be one of self-hate.

Let us consider a health care example in which the person's illness starts to define their identity as being 'unable to'. Imagine a person who develops rheumatoid arthritis. She becomes more and more reclusive, even though the doctors encourage her to be active. However, the arthritis is not just a thing that is happening to her, but becomes a story or narrative of 'what she cannot do'. One needs to understand these narratives of 'I am unable' if the fuller context of her illness and suffering is to be understood. The suffering that comes with an identity of 'I am unable' is essentially given by the painful disjunction between one's felt helplessness and one's hoped for mastery.

Dwelling suffering in the identity dimension: I am an object or 'a thing'

There is a suffering experience that is the consequence of being identified by self or others as 'a thing' or an object. The terrible restriction of this may be felt in different ways: the nauseous anxiety of being turned into something or someone else, the inner scream of 'who one is' being deformed. Here it is almost as if something deep inside oneself knows that its essence is being injured. Some psychologists have called the objectification of self a form of 'soul murder' or 'soul suicide' (Shengold, 1998; Sinason, 2011). This uncanny awareness of being 'pinched' into 'being what I am not' can be perpetrated in many different ways. One may become the brunt of other people, even those whom one loves, who may excessively define one through judgement, in a sense telling one either forcefully or subtly about the kind of 'person' one should become. Or one may engage in the kind of self-betrayal that enacts a self that is manufactured and unsupported. Here, one begins to tread a path where one can no longer find oneself; a person may feel lost, depersonalised or 'unreal'. The suffering of identity as a thing or an object is subject to all the potential injuries of being nothing more than what is measured, and the way that it is measured and compared. The pain of this is in a deep feeling of being unacceptable as one is, unloved. One is then unable to rest in a sense of meaningful personal identity, and one does not feel at home in 'one's own skin'. There is a vicious circle to the way that this painful sense of self as 'object' can become self-perpetuated; there may be a relentlessness to the kind of self-forgetting that occurs with identifying with an image of oneself that is thing-like. One may start to prop up this 'thing-like identity' in different ways, trying to dwell as that, resigning oneself to the contracted horizons of this particular self-image. It may then feel as if something central to oneself is 'at stake'. In a sense this is true, as an 'ontological insecurity' (Laing, 1960/2010) is perpetually announced by the futile unworkability of securing a self as a thing. The 'self as thing' or object can never feel fulfilling, nourishing or peaceful because one's deepest self knows that it cannot accept this state of affairs as 'who one is'.

Imagine an example in which a person's identity becomes defined by their diagnosis in a 'thing-like way'. Here, one may give in to the objectified ways one is being categorised by either the illness or the health care system. One may then define oneself as a 'statistic' or category of person who's condition and behaviour is determined by the 'thing-like' qualities of what they have become: a sense of the uniqueness and non deterministic possibilities of one's identity may be lost. In such a circumstance a carer needs to be extra vigilant in order to avoid colluding with professional and systemic forces that may conveniently find it easier to simply 'treat' the person by objectifying them, thus treating 'categories' and not people. The suffering that comes with an identity of 'I am an object' is essentially given by a certain kind of injury or pain that comes with being turned into something that betrays a self that is always more than 'a thing'.

Dwelling-mobility suffering in the identity dimension: I am fragmented

There is a fragmented hell of personal identity where 'uselessness' and self-objectification are intertwined. There are different variations of this kind of suffering, but in its most extreme forms, one's sense of self is overcome, even possessed by forces that feel alien or 'other'. A coherent sense of self has become fragmented, but more than this, such fragmented identity also carries with it a sense of personal impotence and lack of agency. This dilemma of having lost both self and power have been mythically characterised in different ways: possession by vampires who suck out one's life blood, joining the realm of the walking dead, whether zombie or ghost-like, being haunted by demon-like forces that threaten to turn oneself into something else. But more than this, in this form of suffering, such mythologised forms of objectification render one weak rather than powerful. There may be a sense of 'brokenness' or a self-destruction that has already happened, a loss of coherence and ability, a sense of helpless absence. In such 'dispossession' of self and personal passivity, one may be vulnerable to other voices, influences, addictions, but at its depth, one's eyes are strangely vacant almost as if no one is there. From outside, one may view such an identity as a tragically spent force, a site where a human struggle has been relinquished. In more everyday variations there may be a dissociation of identity in which different 'selves' are compartmentalised. Here, there is an instability of identity; moods may inexplicably change with shifts in state, and others may comment that it is as if one is more than one person. This intertwined form of identity suffering, although most evocatively and intensely described within the context of mental health problems, is also common in the variations of everyday life, for example in major life transitions where one feels depersonalised and disempowered. When personal identity becomes fragmented in various ways and to various degrees, one may feel the annihilatory anxiety that occurs in the process of one's objectification and diminishment. But tragically, in a further development of this, one may feel numb and 'dead inside', like an automaton that is meaninglessly 'going through the motions'. As such, there is a sense of deficient emptiness where 'nothing matters'.

Let us imagine a necessary life-saving health care regime such as renal dialysis. This is an example of how the challenge of coping with very marginal health care conditions can precipitate the potential fragmentation of identity. One is literally in a situation that announces the living of a life that is increasingly not one's own. One may feel taken over and enslaved by a necessary medical regime. Coping strategies may be developed in which one's inner identity is not too deeply affected, but sometimes, 'being taken over' and objectified in this way can go deep inside, and one's identity becomes fragmented. In this fragmentation there may be a deep resignation. Here, the relentless mood of one's day may be occupied by the dull pain of having to give oneself over completely to this 'machine-like' existence. In such a situation, a carer will be particularly sensitised to this dilemma of objectified and powerless identity. The carer will understand this dilemma as a core source of suffering. There is a danger that, in contexts where curative regimes necessarily take one over, this form of identity suffering becomes invisible. A sense of 'fragmented identity' is essentially constituted by the deep existential character of having succumbed to overwhelming objectifying forces that also make one powerless.

Mobility suffering in the embodied dimension: Stasis and exhaustion

There is a physical suffering that is characterised by the body's inability or lack of desire to move, or a felt sense of impaired or threatened bodily functions. An inability to move can be literally imposed such as in paralysis or in other forms of lack of function. This includes 'being stopped in one's tracks' by physical sensations that warn that 'something is wrong'. However there is also a less literal possibility in which the body feels drained of all energy. In both literal and felt versions of blocked bodily mobility or energy, there is a kind of suffering that is essentially characterised by the dark moods of enforced withdrawal: there is a bodily sense that 'nothing can go forward'. This enforced withdrawal particularly refers to the withdrawal of one's bodily powers and vitalities. Literal variations of the body's inability to move include various forms of weakness or dysfunction such as muscle weakness, impaired speech or memory, forms of dis-coordination, tremor, or any other impairment in movement , or normal bodily functioning. In addition, this can include a panicked awareness of difficulties in breathing, swallowing or any other disruption of vital abilities. All of these literal variations interfere with the power of the body to function smoothly in taken-for-granted-ways, to express itself, or to 'body forth' spontaneously or intentionally. In this form of suffering there is a preoccupation with the body, and the feeling of this can vary from panicked alarm to resigned despair. Less literal variations of suffering in the mobility dimension refer to feelings in which one's 'life force' or sense of 'energy' is depleted. At its extreme there is exhaustion, but other forms of a lack of felt vitality may also include listlessness, loss of libido, ennui, lethargy, feeling drained and fatigued. In all of these variations in which bodily movement and vitality recede, there is, intertwined with this, a closing down of significant existential possibilities. Here, one lacks the energy or mobility to pursue and sustain one's aspirations, and to carry out activities that make one's life projects meaningful.

Imagine a person who is experiencing fatigue because of multiple sclerosis or chronic fatigue syndrome. A carer who is sensitive to the meaning of this kind of mobility suffering will understand something about the dilemma of fatigue for the person: that the person may feel split or divided between listening to the body's desire to withdraw and 'go underground', and the person's existential aspirations that require a 'keeping going' and a 'being on the move'. Understanding this dilemma, the carer is able to support the person in such a way that does not collapse into either overemphasising the need for only rest (emphasising a 'sick role'), or on the other hand, over-emphasising a requirement to fit into cultural expectations of activity and vitality (emphasising only a productive role). Rather the carer will help the person to find ways to achieve a balance between the anonymous insistence of one's natural rhythms (in which the body-object participates) and one's everyday desires and existential aspirations. In essence, suffering as a sense of stasis or exhaustion refers to the sense of a body that just cannot support life's desires and meaningful projects.

Dwelling suffering in the embodied dimension: Bodily discomfort and pain

There is a physical suffering that is characterised by bodily discomfort and pain. Here, it is very difficult to simply dwell or feel at home in one's body because of a very palpable sensation that something is wrong. Parts of the body or the body as a whole announces a state of affairs that demands attention. Body parts, isolated sensations, or the whole body 'calls out' as an object of focus in discomfort or pain. The everyday body in well-being, lived as a background that is almost an 'invisible' or 'silent' presence, becomes 'visible' and 'unquiet' in discomfort and pain: bodily well-being is ruptured. This dis-ease, 'against well-being', has an insistent quality, a demanding call for attention and a need for relief, for comfort. One's world contracts to the uncomfortable body or injury and this tends to interrupt all other projects or horizons of meaning, colouring all experience. There are a number of variations of this kind of bodily discomfort that include nausea, irritation, itchiness, tenderness, ache, dizziness, feeling faint or 'woozy', or any other physical sensations of soreness, restlessness or injury. In all this, there may be variations in levels of predictability or unpredictability, persistence, intensity, range and the extent of involvement of body or body parts. People describe many diverse qualities that are not easy to measure or differentiate. So, multiple metaphors are often resorted to, which indicate different kinds and levels of felt wrongness: pulling, penetrating, dragging, grinding, burning, searing, squeezing, gnawing and so on. At its most extreme, pain can become so overwhelming that deep protective strategies of the body take over, and consciousness is lost. Examples of this kind of embodied suffering in health care are many and obvious. But the essence of bodily pain and discomfort is in its experience rather than in our present state of medical knowledge about its physical cause. A carer who honours this profoundly experiential nature of pain or discomfort will not simply dichotomise this experience as either psychological or physical but will always approach the experience in its complexity.

Dwelling-mobility suffering in the embodied dimension: Painful closing down

In principle one can experience physical pain without loss of literal mobility or lack of energy. Conversely, one can experience a loss of literal mobility or lack of energy without experiencing physical pain. However in many circumstances, physical pain arises together with interference or lack of function and/ or with a felt sense of depletion of one's energies. In the body's 'painful or uncomfortable closing down' there is a whole spectrum of suffering, which 'phases in and out'. A person may even enter a 'twilight' world of semi-consciousness in which one feels in a dream-like state that may be described as a 'painful nightmare' of disorientation. In its most extreme variation, such bodily suffering may feel 'unspeakable' in that there are few shared words that can indicate the convergence of both extreme discomfort/ pain and extreme 'closing down' of bodily functions. This is difficult to imagine at its depth, but in some respects, there is an intertwining of pain or discomfort, exhaustion, inability to move and depletion. In essence, in this kind of suffering, there is a felt sense of 'the body closing down' or being overwhelmed in uncomfortable, painful, disintegrating or depleted ways.

The need to care for a wide spectrum of sufferings

So far, beginning in the seamlessness of the lifeworld, we have described eighteen emphases of suffering and attempted to indicate some potential directions for caring practices. However, we do not mean to prescribe these practical directions in an instrumental way. Rather, we are proposing that this framework for understanding can serve as a sensitising resource to guide humanly sensitive care. As in the existential theory of well-being outlined in the previous chapter, the experiential possibilities of suffering should also not be understood in a solely deterministic way as if certain conditions will always inevitably lead to certain suffering experiences. Thus as before, the conditions for suffering such as economic, political, institutional, social, or illness-related, may provide a context for suffering (and either add to or alleviate suffering), but such literal contexts can never fully explain the nature of the suffering. Suffering has its roots in existential depths that always exceed literal causes or explanations, and further, cannot be fully reduced to these causes or explanations.

In taking a phenomenological approach, it has been our aim to describe these eighteen kinds of suffering descriptively, from 'within' the lifeworld, rather than coming to any judgement or value of suffering 'from outside'. We note that suffering can be productive or unproductive depending on its context and circumstance. Experiencing and working with suffering is part of human life and human development. We live between suffering and well-being, just as we live between sky and earth (between freedoms and limits: 'freedom-wound'; Todres, 2007). But the ways that we respond to suffering are telling.

Our view is that an understanding of the eighteen emphases of suffering is important for caring for two reasons: first, it provides a wide descriptive vocabulary that goes beyond signs and symptoms and indicates all the ways that the experience of suffering is connected to all aspects of one's life. Such a language for a spectrum of sufferings may provide a deeper and wider knowledge base by which to care in humanly sensitive ways. But second, an understanding of suffering empowers a crucial capacity that is the source and essence of caring: empathy. A meaningful understanding of suffering can provide empathic power. Such an understanding of suffering reveals the human vulnerabilities that we all share and it therefore announces some of the deepest ways in which humans can have 'a feel' for one another. It is this empathic 'feel' for one another that constitutes a participative form of knowing and without which care would be merely theoretical, abstract or 'only technical'.

We would like to acknowledge that this strong link between caring, empathy and suffering has a longstanding philosophical and disciplinary history. Within existential philosophy, particularly the work of Kierkegaard (cited in Bretall, 1973), there is an emphasis on anxiety and existential despair. Within nursing, the writings of Katie Eriksson (2006, 2007) have been helpful in articulating different contexts and conditions for suffering. For example, she describes how suffering can be existential, can be related to illness, and can even be brought about iatrogenically by poor or neglectful forms and systems of care. Beyond this, other writers have considered other kinds and conditions of suffering such as social suffering, economic suffering, and psychological suffering (Kleinman, Das & Lock, 1997).

However, in relation to caring, we feel that it is most important to keep a felt sense alive of how suffering connects human being to human being. It is this 'shared vulnerable heritage' that forms one of the core foundations of our common humanity, and as we shall cover in the next section, strikes at the heart of the capacity to care.

8 An illustration of well-being as dwelling-mobility

Older peoples' experiences of living in rural areas

In this chapter we would like to show how our well-being theory can widen professional perspectives with regard to situations of vulnerability and deficit in such a way as to offer deeper and more fundamental resources to people. This resource-oriented approach is one that wishes to acknowledge multiple sources of well-being and how access to these additional resources can be helpful in situations of suffering.

Conventional or traditional discourses about the challenges of becoming older often focus on social isolation and increasing bodily vulnerability. We acknowledge that this social and physical emphasis is important and everything possible should continue to be done to try to support older people and to alleviate problems of social isolation and physical/health difficulties. However, beginning in the lifeworld, we will show that well-being, as a kind of 'homecoming' or 'at-homeness', is not just given by social or bodily conditions, but can be intimately experienced in the context of one's deeper connection to the natural world and its rhythms. In this regard, using the perspectives of older people, we would like to tell a story of how the natural world became intimately personal for older people and how such inter-connectivity became their 'bigger story' of well-being, together with their 'social story' and their 'bodily story'. Thus for well-being, the social context is never alone; the bodily context is never alone; all the dimensions of the lifeworld can only be seen 'rhizomatically' as always mutually influential. Here we report on a phenomenological study where a focus on the meaning of mobility expanded to deeper themes concerning elders' well-being; a kind of spatial well-being connected to a sense of 'being at home' in the richly textured places and storied landscapes within which they lived.

A phenomenon that arose unexpectedly out of a larger study

This study that we report here is part of a large-scale research collaboration between five universities, which focused on older peoples' participation in rural civic society. The interdisciplinary study, funded by 'Research Councils UK' was broad ranging and divided into a number of sub studies (work packages) that pursued particular emphases such as, involvement in leisure and cultural activities, contributions to rural community capital, and issues of identity and diversity. This overarching study, called 'Grey and Pleasant Land?' (Hennessey et al., 2012) drew on expertise from a number of different disciplines (geography, social science, psychology, economics) and employed a range of research methodologies. Our phenomenological study was part of a work package that was concerned with the mobility and transport needs of older rural people (Shergold, Parkhurst & Musselwhite, 2012). Within this work package we were interested in the potential insights that a phenomenological approach could contribute to both the conceptualisation and study of older peoples' mobility experiences.

Beginning in the lifeworld, some alternative research questions arose that concerned the meaning of transport, the meaning of mobility and the sense of place experienced by older people living in rural areas. By focusing on the meaning of mobility, and what the meaning of mobility implies for transport, we wished to show how asking a more existential question concerning the spatial dimension of the lifeworld, could perhaps result in some novel insights about *what transport is for* in the everyday lives of older people in rural areas. As we engaged in this open-ended questioning, some interesting insights emerged that we had not fully anticipated. We found that the descriptions we were eliciting from older research participants, although answering some specific interesting questions relevant to transport, also elicited descriptions about their experiences of well-being and place that went far beyond the narrower concern of mobility in itself or transport in itself. This emergent wider concern revealed that the transport needs of older people living in rural areas could not be meaningfully understood without understanding their well-being priorities, the kinds of movement that constituted well-being, and how this related to their feeling of 'at-homeness' in their rural environment. Because of the emergence of this more complex picture, this present chapter will first outline the findings from our planned phenomenological topic, namely, *the meaning of mobility*. But we then follow this with a focus on some unanticipated findings that illustrate the relationship between well-being and a sense of place, and how well-being as a kind of 'homecoming' or 'at-homeness' is not just given by social or bodily conditions but can be intimately experienced in the context of one's deeper connection to the natural world and its rhythms. We came to call this second emergent phenomenon: *rural living as a portal to well-being in older people*.

We now describe our methodological approach which is phenomenological in orientation and follow this by explicating aspects that are revelatory of two phenomena: a) *the meaning of mobility for rural elders*, and b) *rural living as a portal to well-being in older people*.

Our phenomenological study

At the beginning, we pursued an appetite for entering the *phenomenological attitude* in order to delineate our phenomenon and phenomenological research questions. This involved a sense of caution about the ways 'mobility' had been defined from various disciplinary and professional perspectives. This phase resulted in a focus on the meaning of mobility for people and the formulation of 'experience-near' questions that allowed older people to speak of the meaning of 'traversing space', or not, in relation to their everyday lives.

We wished to get close to the lifeworlds of older people living in rural areas in South West England and Wales by devising an interview that explored their everyday life, and the significance of traversing space through movement, however this movement occurred. We wanted to provide older people with maximum opportunities and possible ways to tell us about their 'traverse of space'. This required setting up an interview situation that was open enough to prompt them to talk about significant places that they go to, the meaning of going to those places, why they went to those places, and what they valued about the environments in which they lived and moved. This concern, guided by lifeworld and existential sensibilities was thus much broader than the narrower question of transport and transport 'needs'. It was our overall aim to seek out older peoples' descriptions of variations of all the possible dimensions of rural living in relation to what was important or meaningful to them. Sensitised by an existential view that humans live not just in actualities but in their possibilities, we were interested in, not only the empirical events of the places that were significant to them, but all the possible ways in which they could achieve the purpose of movement. This included literal movement and non-literal movement such as virtual forms of movement and imaginative forms of movement. We were not defining these alternatives in advance but wanted to engage with our research participants in such a way that it did not close them off from talking about these possibilities in whatever ways they wished to.

We undertook ten in-depth phenomenological interviews with rural elders in their own homes in Wales and South West England. These interviews were between one hour and three hours long. The sample of participants was selected according to the following criteria:

1. Older people who were well and who had access to transport.
2. Older people who were well and who had limited access to transport.
3. Older people who were experiencing health difficulties to such an extent as to restrict their mobility.
4. Older people who could not leave their homes.

We sampled from a list of volunteers who where survey participants of the much larger study (Hennessey et al., 2012), of which our study was a part. These volunteers had agreed to follow-up interviews as part of a survey exploring 'Connectivity in older people in rural areas' (Curry & Fisher, in press). Ethical approval of our particular study was gained from the University of Western England Ethics Committee. Potential interviewees were contacted by letter. If older people (age range 65–98 years) wished to participate in our phenomenological work, they were invited to telephone us and we then made arrangements to visit them in their own home. Interviews were undertaken on a one-to-one basis with the authors (but sometimes with couples), and were recorded digitally. Interviews focused on what it is was like to live in the rural place of their residence. The interview also explored 'must-do's', for example, visits to nearby places for shopping; 'have-to's', for example, post office visits to collect a pension or medical appointments; and 'want-to's', an exploration of the desires of older people. The range of questions were developed to allow us to understand a) the meaning of transport in people's lives and b) the meaning of mobility within the context of rural space. We started off with a very broad open-ended question: Can you describe what is it like to live in this rural area and your experience of getting around? This was then followed up by further prompts regarding the meaning and qualities of different kinds of places for them, how they got to them, and what they did if they could not travel. Table 8.1 provides examples of the range of further prompts:

The interviews were audio recorded and transcribed. Our analysis was phenomenological in orientation. We first read each transcript with a view to understanding the integrity of what the transcript indicated as a whole; this understanding served as a holistic meaningful reference and background understanding within which the various parts and detailed meanings of the interview could be understood. We then re-read each transcript identifying changes in meaning and marked these as discrete 'meaning units', which we would each consider in its own right in terms of what it could discretely reveal in relation to the phenomenon we were initially interested in. In the first case: *the meaning of mobility;* and in the second emergent case: *rural living as a portal to well-being in older people.*

We then transformed the language of each of these specific meaning units into more general expressions about the essence of that meaning (transformed meaning unit). We give two examples here of how we transformed a meaning unit in the person's own language to a transformed meaning unit that uses a more essential or general language (see Table 8.2):

The next phase of the analysis involved comparing the transformed meaning units across all interview cases and clustering the most essential

Table 8.1 Example interview questions

- Could you describe an example of going to a place that is a particularly enjoyable place for you?
- How would you get to that place that is particularly enjoyable for you?
- If you can't get to such a place, is there anything that you could do that feels similar?
- Can you describe an experience of places or experiences that you would still really like to see or go?
- Can you describe experiences of places that you like to go on an everyday basis?

Table 8.2 Meaning unit transformed to essential language (transformed meaning unit)

Meaning unit	Transformed meaning unit
We make a point of using the bus. If I do not use it I am losing. Know what I mean? So we try to use the bus at least once a week. It is why we really want to support the bus service. (We have lost the local Post Office).	They make a goal of using the bus as a way to make contributions to supporting the service so that it can be sustainable.
If you are depressed, climb a mountain. [Looking out of his window] I've got the Black mountain range looking up over there, as I said I can see through the gap, right through the Pen Y Fan – the highest point of the Brecon Beacons – which is 30 miles away and I know all the people over there, I know exactly what it is like all around there because I drive there most months	There is a feeling of being uplifted and a sense of familiarity that is carried with him as he looks across to the areas he travels and knows well.

meanings that cohered through all the examples of our interviewees' experiences. After this analysis we wrote an integrated description of the phenomenon that synthesised all the various meanings into 'a whole' so that the phenomenon could be viewed as an essential structure. This description was supplemented by elaborating on its meaning and possible variations, for example, the kinds of mobility that were talked about, what rural space meant for people, what well-being entailed in these circumstances, and so on.

Consistent with the openness of a phenomenological study, a further phenomenon emerged that was significant enough to be named in its own right as a further foundational concern of our interviewees. We have delineated this emergent phenomenon as: *rural living as a portal to well-being in older people*. We now describe our findings of our two phenomena. First, we describe the *meaning of mobility* sensitised by the "continuum of mobilities" (Parkhurst et al., 2012). Second, we describe the essential structure of *rural living as a portal to well-being in older people*.

Findings

The meaning of mobility for older people in rural areas

Essentially the meaning of mobility emerged as a more complex existential and broader phenomenon than the meaning of transport as conventionally defined. A broader phenomenon of 'spatial mobility' emerged from our study. Although including the instrumental concerns and technologies of transport, at its most essential level, spatial mobility was experienced by our sample as *any of the possible ways that people achieve personal life activities where the traverse of space is normally relevant.* We found a number of ways in which participants expressed their traverse of space in meaningful ways, whether literally or not, whereby personal life activities are achieved. Four kinds of mobility that articulated the range of experiences in our phenomenological study emerged from this analysis. Once we were sure about the experiential distinctiveness of these four phenomena, we engaged with our interdisciplinary colleagues in the spirit of a more dialogical moment, in order to name these four kinds of mobility in a way that made sense in this interdisciplinary context (Parkhurst et al., 2012). The existence of three of the phenomena has also been suggested by the literature (e.g. Metz, 2000). We now articulate the four kinds of mobility that emerged:

Literal mobility

This meaning of mobility refers to how older people moved around outside their accommodation in literal ways and this was an important and valued aspect of rural life. Here, a sufficient range of literal transport possibilities were needed, as older people in these rural areas were easily discouraged from traversing space; a threshold of 'a hassle factor' was often experienced. The range of literal transport possibilities were divided into public and private opportunities. Private possibilities of literal transport included 'car owner who drives'; 'car owner whose partner drives'; 'car owner whose friend drives'. The older people in the study greatly valued their access to a private vehicle and this appeared to be related to the felt importance of a kind of control and optionality that was very close at hand. A specific issue in this regard was that these activities could be discouraged by general parking problems, lack of disabled parking facilities, and in situations when commuting to busy towns, a lack of 'park & ride' facilities in some cases. The public transport used by our sample concentrated mainly on commercial bus travel. Volunteer bus services were used when available, and less frequently, trains. It did not take much for our interviewees to feel sufficiently inconvenienced by public transport to the extent that they avoided its use. This sense of significant inconvenience to the degree of non use, did not just occur due to health considerations. Problems with timetables, infrequency of service (daily and weekly), transit connections with long waits, poor disabled access, and the need to carefully plan and negotiate trips (such as hospital appointments), were all described as barriers to the unambivalent embrace of available public transport. On the other hand, as a balance to this inconvenience, there were some clear indications in which older people actively transcended or tolerated these inconveniences for three main reasons:

1. 'Civic conscience', which is characterised by a need to express a solidarity with other members of the community where rural services are being threatened. For example, a couple who have a car, where the husband drives, made a point of using the bus at least once a week: 'if we don't

use it, we will lose it'. This civic conscience was particularly evident with regard to voluntary and pre-bookable bus services, which were perceived as a more personalised bus service.

2. A variation of this is the sense that such transport should be used because, even if older people have current private transport options, they may need public services in the future ("that person who cannot drive will one day be me").

3. Aesthetic considerations, in which older people have the leisure of time, as well as the desire to relax and enjoy countryside views and the conviviality of meeting others on the bus. In essence, it appeared that a significant feature of the instrumental transport choices made concerned not so much the factual availability of transport but its 'goodness of fit' with its convenience and pleasure: life was considered too short to excessively disrupt a 'sense of flow' when making the effort to go places.

Virtual mobility

This meaning of mobility refers to how the purposes of mobility are achieved in an alternative way without significant personal literal movement, either through others or through technology. The variations of virtual mobility refer to a) new and emerging technologies and b) help from others in which the 'outside world' comes in. Technology that affords virtual mobility includes the use of the internet, *Skype*, and webcam to facilitate contact, mostly with family, as an alternative to achieving personal contact through travel and literal mobility: "We have got a webcam so we use the internet and she (grandchild) phones us and we phone back twice a week". Land line and mobile telephones are also used for this purpose, mostly with family. Internet shopping, in which both essential supplies (food), as well as specialist purchases, were considered to be a valuable alternative to literal shopping. A couple who adjusted quickly to rural living partly because they were helped through internet shopping commented: "There are no shops other than the farm shop. We do quite a lot on the net. It helps you get on and not do too much. We can have food and stuff delivered." Another form of virtual mobility refers to help from others. Here, friends, neighbours, professional carers, and services such as meals on wheels, were all cited as ways in which 'the outside world comes in' as an alternative to the need to travel for 'want to' activities and 'have to' activities. Virtual mobility in both its guises, as technological aid and interpersonal aid, were highly valued, not just as essential to people with ill health, but often preferred because of its relative lack of cost and *reach* as balanced against the perceived inconvenience of literal travel.

Imaginative mobility

This meaning of mobility refers to how mobility is achieved in an alternative way without literally moving *by psychological means* through imaginative activities that provide a sense of meaningful spatial engagement, and which achieves a similar psychological outcome to that which would have been achieved through literal movement. This can at times be spontaneous, and at other times, can manifest as 'intentional' or planned for. This form of mobility, as an alternative to literal mobility, is particularly valued by older people whose potentials for both literal mobility and virtual mobility recede (either due to increasing physical limitations, ill health, or lack of desire). The variations consist of any ways in which people extend their sense of connectedness to, and meaningful engagement with, life activities that were previously addressed by literal mobility. This does not involve a simple replacement of the 'old' established activity (e.g. "going to the pub to meet longstanding friends") but rather involves something that is more complex that we found evidence for, that is, the achievement of a different but allied experience through other means (e.g. reminiscing about longstanding friends and stories with visitors and through photographs). Other descriptions of experience that indicated imaginative mobility included the 'portals' of television and reading, listening to and playing music, being in close proximity and caring for pets and wildlife, access to views of the landscape, close proximity to nature, gardens, and responding experientially to the changes and rhythms of the seasons. These portals to imaginative mobility were found to be significant aids by which, as an older person's literal mobility possibilities receded, imaginative pathways were opened up to either a life that is possible or a life that was being held onto. One older women confined to one room has found a fulfilling alternative to literal movement by imaginatively listening to music and engaging the scenes that it conjures up from the past: "its something I knew a long time ago-dancing and the happy times then, . . . the music takes me back there". An older housebound woman who has always been interested in astronomy: "since a little girl I always looked at the moon . . . I have got a telescope, I looked out the other night, you can't miss to see Venus . . . it's the brightest of the stars". She went on to explain: "I love watching the sunsets, by next month it will be rising over there, then it will be over there . . . and I like looking at that".

This is an important 'quality of life' alternative to that which was previously achieved by literal mobility and therefore needs to be considered as part of the spectrum of spatial mobility engagement. This form of mobility meets an intrinsic desire in people to feel that they are moving forward in some sense and are connected to their possibilities.

Potential mobility

This meaning of mobility refers to a situation where the potential to travel is literally available but this availability is sufficient as a fulfilling experience without having to move. Potential mobility thus has characteristics of literal mobility as well as imaginative mobility but combines these in a unique way: the possibility of literal mobility is the foundation for potential mobility but is not actualised; it is not actualised because the mere experience of knowing that it is literally possible is enough of a fulfilling experience, and this fulfilling experience has an imaginative quality. Variations of potential mobility concern a range of mobility choices that are possible but not taken, such as "a trip to the coast or far away." For example, a couple who did not have plans to go anywhere far, explained that they had plans to go to a seaside resort sometime in the future, but it was enough fulfilment for them to feel the potential mobility of this as an option: "It's not a must-do, it's just a feeling that it could be nice to explore a bit more of Cornwall".

We would like to acknowledge that these four kinds of spatial mobility and its variations may be common to all people whether in rural situations or not. However our data and analysis points to two important considerations about becoming older and about rural habitat that signifies something distinctive: a) for older people, virtual, imaginative and potential mobility become significantly more important as alternatives to literal mobility either because of health reasons or because their motivations for movement become reprioritised, b) the older people living in a rural habitat evaluate their motivated engagements with spatial mobility in terms of a value of convenience in relation to the specific desire to 'dwell' in their 'home-like' rural environment.

Rural living as a portal to well-being in older people

As described in the phenomenon: *the meaning of mobility,* the older people in our study painted a picture of how the traverse of space in various aspects of their lives was important to them. They described everyday life in 'moving around' terms, how they used transport and the mobility opportunities available. But more than this, they included descriptions of what was important to them in sustaining their quality of life: they spoke of the places that they *needed* to go to as well as the places that they *desired* to go to, and how they achieved the purpose and outcomes of mobility without always literally traversing space. But also, they spoke about rural life, the significance of place, the significance of nature, and the significance of heritage connections. They described a temporal rhythm and how they personally fitted into all of this. This included thoughts they had about getting older, their values and how their values had changed, and how the landscape and nature were significant for their experience of well-being. In our presence to all of this, what appeared to announce itself, was that a particular kind of well-being in relation to rural place was a significant enough phenomenon in its own right, and that this called for deeper analysis and articulation. We now articulate this phenomenon that we call: *rural living as a portal to well-being in older people.*

Essential structure of the phenomenon: Rural living as a portal to well-being in older people

A certain kind of well-being related to rural place emerged as an essential phenomenon. This connection between well-being and rural place was constituted by two interrelated experiences: the importance of dwelling and slowing down at this stage of our participants' lives; and the importance of a 'rich textured locale' for the well-being of rural older people.

The importance of dwelling and slowing down

There were notable findings that suggested an increased interest in what we are calling 'dwelling' as an emphasis. The term 'dwelling' refers to an overall 'willingness to be here' and even an increasing preference for a kind of less active lifestyle that is nourished by a sense of 'at-homeness' within the rural landscape. Related experiences expressed in this connection were those of a preference for peace, privacy, beautiful natural views, 'being in nature', being far from the crowd, and generally a life that reflects less goal-oriented 'being there'. When literal mobility opportunities recede there is often less of a sense of regret because of the welcome emphasis on 'at-homeness'. It is in this context that both virtual mobility and imaginative mobility become important alternatives to literal mobility as well-being resources. There were two variations that constituted the motivation to dwell and slow down; we have called these: 'prompted to dwell' and 'choice to dwell'. Being prompted to dwell refers to situations in which a person's life circumstances, such as ill health or carer responsibilities resulted in a prompt to reconsider their life's priorities, and how a slower life may be easier for them. In this regard one man said: "we wanted a bit more peace because I had cancer." A person who cares for his wife commented: "In my life as a carer my home is very important. I can't imagine living in my previous situation. It would be quite claustrophobic." He now enjoys the open vistas of the forest and rhodo-dendrons, the typical old English countryside, and the wilderness there, "particularly at night time". The variation that we have called 'choice to dwell' refers to situations in which there is more freedom to consider their life's priorities, often accompanied by fulfilment in being close to the natural world. But often, new developmental stages brought on by ageing (such as retirement) may result in the wish for a simpler, more peaceful life. An example is given by a man who decided to move to a more rural situation because of the desire for greater peace: "I go and sit out there and you know . . . nobody, no sirens and things like cars. I sit out there – there is a little summer house – [I go there] especially in the Spring or Autumn when it is not hot." Another woman indicated: "it's nice listening to the birds and seeing all the trees and the flowers come out, and all that and looking at the sky and the sun coming up or going down". Further, a couple who knew very well what is in a thirty mile radius of their home, and whose garden is very important to them said: "It's like being on your own world, nothing we actually need . . . and we have the roses".

The importance of a rich textured locale for the well-being of rural older people

There were notable findings that suggested an intimate knowledge and valuing of their local rural vicinity as a 'storied' place that was rich with personal, communal and landscaped history, and which gave the immediate locale 'a human face'. The well-being possibilities of this textured locale generally begins outside the front door and its horizon stretches to include places necessary for day-to-day requirements (such as post office, doctor's surgery, local shop), as well as places that are important for older peoples' sense of enjoyment usually related to their preference for rural living (such as garden centres, heritage sites, coastal walks, and familiar places that have personal historical significance for them). An older woman who can't go out because of illness spoke of all the places nearby that are full of stories for her: ". . . like the goat who used to live down there . . . she would not let women into the field . . . but a man could go into the garden . . . the goat would not eat anything else but if panties were on the line she would pinch them". She also spoke about various places that have changed in meaning over time: "The canals remind me of the past, we had no money. If we could not catch a rabbit, or the hens didn't lay, we did not have enough food . . . we had no money but we so enjoyed everything here". Another woman, also housebound talked of how she sits outside and can imagine what it is like further afield: "there is a dingle down there and there is a tunnel up the other end and there is a tunnel of trees." She loves the trees. The cherry tree reminds her of the man with the sheep dog and the times when she went wandering in the woods. A man spoke of how he had got to know this landscape he lived in through a long history of having moved through it: "I have travelled all the country lanes and everywhere." He knows all the places where the forest has receded and when. The notion of the richness of 'textured locale' is epitomised by a comment from one of our interviewees. An older man was visited by his granddaughter in the rural countryside. She looked around and exclaimed "Granddad, you live in the middle of nowhere!" To which he replied, "No, I live in the middle of everywhere"'.

When literal mobility opportunities recede there is often a need to draw on their knowledge of this textured locale and the mobility resources offered within this locale. The importance of a rich textured locale for well-being has within it a number of different nuances that emerged from our analysis of elders who've grown up and lived in the area all their lives, and those elders who had moved into the area, often to retire. There are some important distinctions between these elders: Long-standing elders of the area particularly valued the depth of *this* storied place in which they had participated in for a lifetime; they were aware of the story of the place that preceded them but had also built up over time a rich personal history that arose out of their living there through the seasons and the changes. The following quote is from an older man who had seen his grandchildren grow up there, who has been to many weddings and funerals, and who has a community of friends and farmers who are connected to his past work life: "I am part of the community because I get things done . . . I planted a tree that will be there for another 100 years . . . I am chasing my ancestors at the moment who lived not really far away. Most of them were born ten miles away . . . so the family name will go on . . ." Those elders who had moved into the area also shared some sense of this historical connection to the place, but with two variations:

1. This group generally came to the rural place because of their desire and/ or need to slow down. For example a couple moved from London about 10 years ago and now live in a rural parish of 400 people: "after London we came here for a better life. We felt we were getting the rush, the hub bub". Another gentleman commented: "Our dream was the rural living . . . in the country you get four distinct seasons, you know, . . . you get the Winter".
2. This group were also often attracted to a particular place because of a past historical significance that was personally meaningful to them. For one couple, a personal historical connection to the area was important. They referred to their personal connection to the area by saying: "This old house, a ruin really. I have known it since a toddler and we go there regularly . . . we have always loved it, and there is a fountain which is fantastic to see".

The rhythms around us: Well-being wisdom from rural elders

We believe that there are some unanticipated implications of our study for understanding the nature of well-being. The rural elders in our study confirmed some of the emphases of the dwelling-mobility theory of well-being in that the experience of 'at-homeness' or 'dwelling' is central to experiential well-being. But these rural elders provided two particularly important insights: a) that a 'storied' connection to our natural world and its rhythms may be just as important for well-being as the social or bodily conditions for well-being b) that in our present culture the value of mobility as a source of well-being may have been overemphasised, and that the value of dwelling for well-being may have been obscured.

The storied connection to our natural world as a resource for well-being

Rural elders in this phenomenological study all independently and spontaneously spoke of the richness of their 'rural place' as a source of 'at-homeness', dwelling and well-being. We were moved to call this dimension of their 'living in' and 'living with' these personal rhythms of the natural world, 'textured locale'. 'Textured locale' clearly announced itself as a crucial 'portal' or pathway to well-being. Such rural places thus emerged as a liminal space that connected personal meanings to a natural world that is before and beyond them; such meaningful places were not just 'spatial' but temporal as well; they were always 'wet through' with history and heritage. At its depths this connectivity was not separate from what well-being could be: an intimate continuity between self and broader 'natural' ecological contexts that speak with a 'human face'. This phenomenon, which we called *rural living as a portal to well-being in older people*, has some resonance with some anthropological descriptions of traditional societies' embeddedness in what they call 'an environing earth' and a participatory 'place centred' living (Abram, 1996). Such anthropological and ecological perspectives often include arguments about how older people in these ancient cultures had a crucial and respected role to play in connecting people to their past and to 'textured locales' that supported them. In our current and modern day study we thus heard our rural elders calling us back from a decontextualised discourse about environment and mobility needs to a well-being discourse in which 'at-homeness' did not appear to be separate from the rural rhythms of place. And in our view, it is not a matter of chance that it is older people that are well placed to remind us of the importance of 'at-homeness'.

This message about a sense of place as a resource for well-being is a remedy to much current discourse that overemphasises social inclusion as a source of well-being. Here, we would like to re-emphasise the possibility of our connectivity to the natural world or place as a source of well-being. We wish to do this not because we would like to deny the importance of either the social dimensions of well-being or even its physical bodily dimensions, but because the 'place dimension' of well-being (spatial well-being) may be at risk of becoming an obscured perspective. This empirical study thus appears to confirm the relevance of the spatial dimension for well-being, especially when possibilities for some of the other well-being resources are in recession. This is not to say that the other dimensions of well-being such as temporal well-being, interpersonal well-being, embodied well-being, and emotional well-being are not important but that this phenomenological study points to findings that emphasise the value of spatial well-being.

An overemphasis in our culture on mobility as a source of well-being

If our phenomenological study moved towards an emphasis on dwelling, well-being and textured locale, what are the implications of these findings for our initial aim of understanding the mobility needs of rural elders? Our phenomenological lifeworld orientation resulted in findings that suggested that one cannot understand the meaning of mobility for older people living in rural areas (what was important to them about the need and wish to traverse space) without understanding how this is in play with dwelling (their sense of 'at-homeness' in their rich textured locale). In other words, the meaning of mobility is intertwined with the meaning of dwelling and cannot be considered alone; the value of feeling at home or otherwise is a crucial context for understanding what mobility means to older people. Dwelling, or the 'willingness and ease' of being here, of residing here, of being in a rich textured locale, this rural space, with many meanings, histories and communal significances, becomes particularly important for the older people in our study. The implication of 'an increased interest in dwelling' is that the need for mobility became less important as a primary source of well-being. Life became less goal-oriented. This is not to say that mobility as an option and possibility is unimportant for well-being. But more, that our rural elders were reminding us about a more dialectical phenomenon as a source of well-being, namely the *rhythm* of dwelling and mobility. This reminder about this rhythm made us wonder whether in our current cultural context of fast moving aspirations and targets, mobility as a value is overemphasised, and dwelling as a value may be obscured as a legitimate source of well-being. In our study, the rural elders were speaking about this rhythm in relation to rural life. We wish to acknowledge however that this rhythm of mobility and dwelling can occur in other spatial contexts such as a city (Hillman, 2006). In this study it was just that living rurally seemed to provide a powerful reminder of the value of dwelling. So, our older people appear to be telling us that we need to honour both dimensions, in play with one another. So at the end of this study we discovered our participants as mentors who were teaching us about a possible split in our culture. In calling us back to this rhythmical play, and to the well-being intimacies of living within 'textured locales', they have, in our view, brought a potentially healing voice forward from out of the shadows.

Part III

Developing the capacity to care

This section provides a meditation on the question of 'what it takes' to develop the capacity to care within an academic, professional and personal context. Etymologically, the word 'capacity' is partially derived from the Latin term '*capax*', which indicates: 'that can contain' or 'able to hold much' (*Online Etymological Dictionary*). In a contemporary context, 'capacity' is defined as 'the ability or power to do or to understand' (*Oxford English Dictionary*). This concern with the 'capacity to care' has led us in our writings to a number of interrelated issues which are focused on the kinds of epistemologies, research methodologies, pedagogies and practice development approaches that heal any split between knowing and feeling. It is within this context that we offer the notion of 'embodied relational understanding'. First, our sensibility includes the wish to show that a certain kind of knowing is conducive to developing the capacity to care, and that within this context, lifeworld-oriented research is valuable. Second, we wish to show the close connectedness between developing the capacity to care and an aesthetic sensibility that is especially opened up by the worlds of the arts and the humanities. Third, we wish to indicate how the capacity to care is constituted by an openness to 'otherness' and difference. Each of the following chapters thus emphasise one or more of these connections, but together provide an existential-phenomenologically informed approach to the places where a certain kind of knowing and a certain kind of feeling are already together at the heart of what caring is. Sometimes we concentrate on the nature of humanly hospitable research methodologies, sometimes on more aesthetic kinds of re-presentation and knowing, and sometimes on the necessary open-hearted rhythm between a certain kind of knowing and a certain kind of 'not-knowing'.

Chapter 9 makes the case for more contemplative forms of knowledge that may helpfully underpin caring practices. This theoretical chapter thus concentrates on epistemological issues.

Within the context of health and social care education, attempts to define 'scholarship' have increasingly transcended traditional academic conceptions of the term. While acknowledging that many applied disciplines call for a kind of 'actionable knowledge' that is also not separate from its ethical dimensions, engagement in the caring professions in particular provides an interesting exemplar that raises questions about the nature and practice of 'actionable knowledge:' how is such knowledge from different domains (the head, hand and heart) integrated and sustained? This chapter outlines some philosophical ideas that may be important when considering the characteristics of the kind of scholarship for caring practices that draw on deep resources for creativity and integration.

First, there is an attempt to clarify the nature of scholarly practice by drawing on Aristotle's notion of '*phronesis*' (practical wisdom). Second, a more meditative approach to the integration of knowledge, action and ethics is highlighted. Finally, its implications for scholarship are introduced, in which scholarly integration may best be served by more contemplative ways of being and thinking. Drawing on Heidegger and Gendlin, we consider the challenges of contemplative thinking for pursuing scholarly practice. We articulate contemplative thinking as an unspecialised mode of being that is given to human beings as an intimate source of creativity. The sense in which unspecialisation can be cultivated and practised is discussed.

In Chapter 10 we are particularly interested in what facilitates the 'heart' of care, that is, the kind of empathic understanding that is required to 'walk a mile in another's shoes'. From an epistemological point of view, this capacity requires an ability to imagine what it may be like to live with various illness conditions.

Here we build on some of the ideas of the previous chapter regarding the kind of knowledge that is particularly relevant to caring practice, but further develop the ways in which qualitative research findings can serve such knowledge. As phenomenological researchers, we have been engaged with the question of how findings from such research can be re-presented and expressed more aesthetically. Such a movement towards a more aesthetic phenomenology may serve the communicative concern to express phenomena relevant to caring practice in ways that appeal to the 'head, hand and heart'. The chapter first offers some thoughts about the complex kind of knowledge relevant to caring that is not only technical or propositional, but actionable and aesthetically moving as well. As previously indicated, we have named this kind of knowledge 'embodied relational understanding', and revisit some of the ideas contributing to this notion. Further, the chapter outlines the development of one way of serving this more aesthetic phenomenology whereby research findings can be faithfully and evocatively translated into empathically impactful expressions. We call this process 'embodied interpretation'. It is guided by an epistemological framework grounded in the philosophies of Gadamer and Gendlin. We finally illustrate the process with reference to the experience of living after stroke, and consider the value of this translational process for professional education and practice.

In Chapter 11 we focus in more depth on the method of 'embodied interpretation', the particular methodology that we have developed to translate qualitative research findings already in the public arena into more evocative forms that may empower the empathic imagination. The chapter contributes to a growing trend in articulating an aesthetic phenomenology that exercises more evocative and poetic forms of writing. Our task is to give ontological weight to our common humanity, thereby facilitating experiences of recognition and 'homecoming'. This developing trend could benefit from Gendlin's philosophy of the body and his practice of 'focusing', which finds words that carry forward the textural dimensions of experience. We briefly illustrate the practice of embodied interpretation with reference to an earlier chapter about caring for a life-long partner with Alzheimer's disease. We conclude that the value of embodied interpretation is that it serves the kind of knowledge that is particularly important in human sciences – it provides understandings that live in ways that touch both 'head' and 'heart'. And, by facilitating such 'touched understandings', research findings can make a difference to the deepening of empathic understanding in readers and practitioners.

Chapter 12 addresses more directly the challenge of integrating knowing, feeling, aesthetic sensibility, embodied practice, and an openness to 'otherness', for the sake of humanly sensitive care. We meditate on this integrative task in relation to what we believe is a crucial phenomenon within the discipline of nursing: that is the phenomenon of 'nursing open-heartedness'. We articulate the central role that 'nursing open-heartedness' may play in guiding caring in complex situations, and use vignettes of everyday nursing life situations to illustrate the following three essential dimensions that constitute 'nursing open-heartedness':

• The infinity of otherness: keeping open the other's difference through a certain kind of 'not knowing'.
• Embodiment: our shared vulnerable heritage.
• Practical responsiveness: embracing the value of the objectified gaze and technology.

Each of these dimensions is philosophically informed by distinctive insights from the work of Heidegger, Levinas and Merleau-Ponty. Further, guided by Gendlin's contributions regarding the nature of embodied understanding, we employ a writing style that attempts to present the nature of 'nursing open-heartedness' as a possible experience rather than as an abstract theory.

The final chapter will offer a coherent synthesis of our distinctive approach to the humanisation of care. We will conclude with a brief overview that provides a conceptual integration of 1) humanisation as a value, 2) well-being and suffering as a focus, and 3) a consideration of how the capacity for care is based on an integration of being and knowing. These three foci help to articulate the thematic unifying narrative of the book namely, caring for well-being.

9 The creativity of 'unspecialisation'

Contemplative knowledge and practical wisdom

Caring may require an epistemological foundation that transcends some of the more recent dichotomies that have tended to overcompartmentalise knowledge into discrete disciplines. This has concurrently coincided with an overspecialisation of professional domains. We argue that the kind of knowledge that needs to be reclaimed for a meaningful humanly sensitive care is holistic and integrative. In this chapter we offer some epistemological considerations by which these notions of holistic knowledge and integrated practice can be clarified.

We thus wish to contribute to an emerging debate about what scholarship means in a changing world where domains of knowledge have become exceedingly complex, in that knowledge is increasingly specialised and raises significant challenges for how these different discourses relate to one another in both theory and practice. Such complexity is particularly highlighted in caring professions such as nursing, midwifery, medicine, psychology, social work and other professions allied to medicine, where immersion in practice has exposed a deep inseparability between knowledge, ethics and action.

Boyer (1990) put forward a model of scholarship that emphasised the integration of a number of scholarly domains including research, teaching and application. In 1999, the American Association of Colleges of Nursing (AACN, 1999) adopted a position statement on scholarship that built on Boyer's work. Riley, Beal, Levi and McCausland (2002) took this further and proposed that such scholarship is setting-related but not setting-dependent, that it is holistic and fluid, and that it combines knowledge, experience, rigour and a service base. In a wide-ranging article, they consider some of the complexities of knowledge-in-action and knowledge-for-action, in which the sources of knowing are intimately intertwined with experience and practice. In this way, Riley et al. (2002) refer to how a very local and situated engagement is relevant to knowledge production: "The intimacy of the relationship is essential; because it provides important information and it is the therapeutic vehicle for applying knowledge" (p. 386).

These ideas draw on a tradition of thought that focuses on forms of applied knowledge (e.g. Benner & Chesla, 1998; Benner, Hopper-Kyriakidis & Stannard, 2010; Carper, 1978; Schon, 1983; Van Manen, 1999b). By emphasising action, service orientation and immersion in practice, this tradition integrates knowing and being (epistemology and ontology), and includes the ethical dimension of the 'good'.

In this chapter, we meditate further on the integration of knowledge, ethics and action and pursue the following goals:

- Locating the separation of the domains of knowledge, ethics and action within a historical context.
- Considering the nature of *'phronesis'* – the kind of knowledge that is already not separate from ethics and action.
- Formulating 'scholarship' as a 'seamless' way of being, rather than the integration of separate domains of knowledge, ethics and action.
- Indicating some directions for promoting a scholarship that draws on more contemplative directions which open up creative, 'unspecialised' possibilities for feeling, thinking and doing. The term 'unspecialised' is developed in relation to Heidegger's thought and expresses a fundamentally human way of being that cannot be objectified and as such is a deep source of creativity.

We conclude by considering whether the creativity of 'unspecialisation' can be practised, and draw on Heidegger and Gendlin as helpful guides.

A conceptual exploration of scholarship for caring practices

Historical context: The 'dignity' and 'disaster' of modernity

In this section we would like to briefly offer one perspective on the gradual specialisation of knowledge. Although there are, of course, many accounts of the fragmentation of knowledge domains (e.g. Habermas, 1990; Taylor, 1985; Weber, 1963), we offer a brief historical analysis that draws on Wilber's (1995) discussion of the postmodern separation of science, art and morality. Understanding modernity and postmodernity as historical phenomena, the first of these can be identified with the project of the enlightenment in which the progress of natural science became a primary source of knowledge, value and justice. The second, postmodernity, refers to a certain epistemological and ethical disillusionment with scientific progress. We acknowledge that particular strands of postmodern thought have been accused of certain excesses of relativism and even narcissism, but also acknowledge other strands within this discourse that emphasise respect for diversity in terms of values and culture as well as the validity of heterogeneous ways of knowing. It is within this distinction between modernity and postmodernity as a historical phenomenon that Wilber (1995) brings together a historical analysis of the sociology of knowledge that began with Weber (1963) and which was pursued further by Taylor (1985) and Habermas (1990). Central to this analysis are the developments of modernity that heralded the differentiation: science, art and morality. This differentiation allowed much progress to take place in the spheres of the sciences, the arts and justice, because each domain could pursue its activities without having to be too contaminated by the concerns of the other. Science was less constrained by aesthetic or ethical concerns, which allowed it to concentrate on the pursuit of knowledge in the objective world. This heralded technological progress in attempts to control the environment and human world. Art, too, became much less classically wedded to morality or to an accurate and knowing portrayal of reality. What Wilber (1995, p. 416) calls the "dignity of modernity" refers to the positive value of modernity, the advantages of creating the space for specialisation, where welcome progress could be made within each domain's own terms, and in accordance with their own logic:

> By the end of the eighteenth century, science, morality and art were even institutionally *differentiated* as realms of activity in which questions of truth (science), of justice (morals), and of taste (art) were autonomously elaborated, that is, each of these *spheres of knowing* [was pursued] under its own specific aspect of validity.
>
> (Habermas, 1990, p. 19, original italics)

Such differentiation, however, poses the question that has become increasingly apparent in our times: how can these different domains become re-integrated? According to Wilber, the disaster of modernity is that these domains, through their specialised paths, have become dissociated from one another: ". . . if the *dignity* of modernity was the differentiation of the Big Three, the *disaster* of modernity would be that it had not yet found a way to *integrate* them" (Wilber, 1995, p. 416). Habermas (1990) has been strident in his criticism of what he called the 'colonisation of the lifeworld' by social engineering, technical approaches to practical life and subjectivity, and the increasing control by 'experts' of political and social life. All this constituted a 'commodification'; to turn into mere commodities the values of life. Habermas (1990) elaborated on how the differentiation of the domains of science, art and morality created a situation of uneven development in these spheres, and how a healing of such dissociation is needed. We are currently scrambling to address the ethics and justice of scientific progress, the art of applied knowledge and the boundaries of art, and the scientific and aesthetic dimensions of law. A metaphorical way to express Wilber's question about integration would be: how do the head (knowing), the heart (ethics) and the hand (the art of action) function as one body? What is this way of being and what are its implications for the meaning of scholarship?

In postmodern times, we cannot simply turn back to a form of simplistic holism in a way that denies specialisation and diversity. However, in honouring differentiation, we can, nevertheless, pursue such differentiated domains through an understanding of the fundamental non-separation of science, morality and the art of action in the way that life *moves*. We may need to make this background much clearer when considering scholarship and so we refer to Aristotle's notion of a way of being in which knowing, doing and valuing are fundamentally inseparable.

The nature of 'phronesis': The kind of knowledge that is already not separate from ethics and action

Polkinghorne (2004) advocates an expanded notion of rationality that can accommodate living situations that are highly specific to their context, that involve the unpredictability of the human realm, and where exceptions to rules often apply: "Effective practices of care require that practitioner actions are decided by their situated and timely judgements" (p. 2). Furthermore:

> Practical choices in situations calling for actions to bring about the human good require a kind of thought that can deal with complex and competing goals and take into account the timing and context of the action, as well as the uniqueness and particular characteristics of the situation and person for whom the action is undertaken.
>
> (Polkinghorne, 2004, p. 21)

In this view, scholarship is tested by the ". . . situations in which we run out of rules" (Brown, 1988, p. 139). So what kind of knowing and way of being is adequate for this task? Polkinghorne refers back to ancient Greece, before the differentiation of the value spheres had taken place, to Aristotle.

Aristotle (1983) distinguished between the kind of deliberations that were appropriate for making things (techne) and those that were appropriate for acting in the human realm. He used the term 'phronesis' to mean a practical wisdom that can address a plurality of values.

> The most characteristic function of a man of practical wisdom is to deliberate well: no one deliberates about things that cannot be other than they are, nor about things that cannot be directed to some end, an end that is a good attainable by action. In an unqualified sense, that man is good at deliberating who, by reasoning, can aim at and hit the best thing attainable to man by action.
>
> (Aristotle, 1983, 1141b 9–14)

The complexity of living situations means that such plurality often results in conflict between values: conflicts such as the good of an individual versus the good of the collective, or conflicts that surround the inherent risks of acting versus not acting when certainty of outcome cannot be guaranteed. The sources of understanding and knowing that are drawn on in such situations are multiple, and are already based on an interwoven fabric of knowing, morality and the art of applied action. Such interwoven 'fabric' is only separated into categories by means of reflection – it is originally a seamless way of being and moving. Polkinghorne sees such a way of being as an expansion of the traditional understanding of rationality; it is intelligent in that it varies with situations, is receptive to particulars, and has the quality of improvisation. Polkinghorne links Aristotle's notion of *phronesis* to a number of current developments in philosophy and psychology that articulate a broader understanding of rationality. We merely wish to indicate these developments in order to acknowledge that there are currently a number of ways to develop a kind of practical wisdom that emphasises the way human beings are embedded in their world.

This broader understanding of rational thinking includes Epstein's (1994) 'experiential thinking', Lakoff and Johnson's (1999) 'embodied rationality' and Gendlin's (1962) notion of the 'felt sense'. These notions resonate deeply with Aristotle's *phronesis*. However, in this paper, we would like to highlight 'empathic imagination' as a kind of practical wisdom of particular relevance to caring practices.

First of all, empathic imagination involves imaginative thinking. Murray (1986) draws on Heidegger to show how this is not simply an imaginary experience, such as imagining being able to fly like Peter Pan; imaginative thinking is more directed in that it may be used to solve complex problems. It is also a participative form of knowing, in that you imaginatively put yourself in a series of scenarios so as to be open to the possibilities of those scenarios. Such thinking is particularly relevant when a unique situation asks you to dwell with the specific complexities of that situation. Imaginatively we see what is *there* and what is *not there* and move forward in time to imagine outcomes and possibilities. In that way, we participatively and imaginatively move in many directions, in a 'rhizomatic' manner, just as a rhizome is a plant with an intricacy of interconnections. In imaginative thinking there is the interconnection between past and future, feeling, thought and situation; a multiplicity of felt connections. Emphasising the difference between generality and particularity, Nussbaum (1990) indicates the complexity of such interconnected, imaginative presence:

> Instead of ascending from the particular to the general, deliberative imagination links particulars without dispensing with their particularity. It would involve, for example, the ability to recall past experiences as one with, as relevant to, the case at hand, while still conceiving of both with rich and vivid concreteness.
>
> (Nussbaum, 1990, p. 78)

As one kind of deliberative imagination, empathic imagination goes further. It brings in an interpersonal focus whereby *the world* of another person is imagined. The phenomenological tradition has been helpful in articulating an approach to understanding others by trying to suspend our own preconceptions and 'taking a walk in another person's shoes'. Developmental psychologists such as Kohlberg (1981) have shown how moral development requires the ability to shift from an egocentric position to one that can see something from another's point of view. Empathic imagination is thus already an interwoven fabric of thinking, ethics and action in that an individual is fundamentally engaged in *being with* and, in some cases, *being for* another as a source of knowledge and action. The meaning of caring is founded on this possibility, with its imagination of what another's world may be like. It provides rich, detailed and context-specific possibilities for knowing and acting. Therefore, it is a form of *phronesis* (practical wisdom) that may be centrally important when considering the meaning of scholarship for caring practices.

Scholarship as a seamless way of being rather than the integration of separate domains of knowledge, ethics and action

Our consideration of the kind of scholarship that is central to caring practices has so far emphasised a kind of integration of knowledge, ethics and action that intimately work together as a coherent movement. For caring practices we have emphasised how this kind of integration is centrally informed by an empathic sensibility that underpins such integration. We would like however to consider further the nature of this kind of integration.

There is a danger in any analysis of 'integration', which is that integration of knowing, ethics and action is achieved by actively *doing* such integration. This often serves to increase the feeling that we are 'in over our heads' (Kegan, 1994), again scrambling to increase our professional life-loads by becoming everything: researchers, teachers, business-fellows and internet junkies perusing the latest evidence. The felt quality of this often constitutes a sense of impending fragmentation rather than a sense of coherence; but the question is: what gets 'dropped out' in all this increased doing?

An alternative view of integration that is more contemplative and less strident is provided by Heidegger (1993b) and is essentially contained in his image of a clearing in the forest. Within this image, once such a clearing has been attained, integration does not have to be actively strived for, because what was thought of as requiring integration (as separate domains) is found to already be there, 'together'. This view of integration suggests an uncovering of what can obscure it rather than an active search to put things together, as if this needs to be achieved through ardour and artifice. Such *uncovering* requires a more contemplative direction and draws on a critique by Heidegger of the spirit of technology, and how this can obscure integrative possibilities as a way of being.

In the 1920s, Heidegger (1927/1962) was already facing fundamental questions about the relationship between the spirit of technology and more foundational issues of being human. He wasn't against technological progress but wanted to strike a note of caution about how the essence of technology is such that it is defining not only the world around us, but also ourselves as objects. Furthermore, he was concerned that as we became increasingly capable of objectifying ourselves in this way, something very important would become obscured – namely our unspecialised capacity of being. Such unspecialised capacity is the place where knowing, ethics and action were never separate. It is rather 'one song' (Todres, 2000a) or a movement that is always unfinished because it is open to the new and is already an interconnection of head, hand and heart; it is the realm of possibility. In this view, integration has always been happening and we only become excessively concerned with integration if it is blocked or if we wish to overly control its direction.

Nurturing the space for such being-possibilities does not mean that nothing is happening. Applying this to a kind of scholarship that is a seamless movement of head, hand and heart would mean that the ongoing learning and opportunities within our professional and personal lives could 'settle'. The importance of 'settling' as a kind of clearing that allows integration to be, does not eradicate the value of pursuing specialised developments or the activity of relating these developments to one another. Rather, it offers some relief that striving in a specialised way is not the only path to productivity – that our unspecialised capacities for being can be productive. As touched on earlier in this paper, this is the place from where integration is already vitally tasted. The question then changes from *how to 'effortfully' achieve a scholarly integration of knowledge, ethics and action*, to *how to bring specialised activities into the spaciousness of being where integration is already 'humming'*. Approaching the question in this way may raise particular challenges for how we support this possibility. The kind of scholarship that attempts to accommodate such a *how* may be best conceptualised as a way of being that needs a different kind of support and permission by our learning and institutional contexts. The challenge is then to recognise such times of settling as a creative resource for seamless knowing-valuing-acting. The feeling-quality of such settling and connecting with this natural integrity may be one of vitality. There may be a certain sense of excitement and coherence as we begin to give space to and trust these possibilities of being. Such a sense of vitality and coherence may also mitigate a feeling of burnout. We consider later how a more contemplative scholarly path can be given permission and supported with reference to Gendlin's philosophy of entry into the implicit. But first we would like to consider the path of contemplation as a way of being that is relevant to scholarship for caring practices.

A contemplative scholarship: Can unspecialisation be practised?

Turner (1994), Van Manen (1999b) and others have indicated the complexity of the notion of 'practice' in relation to pedagogy. In this view, practice is not merely instrumental in the sense of applying pre-determined methodologies, but is rather embedded in ways of being that are pre-reflective and often spontaneous. Does this mean that such practice 'just happens' or is there a way that we can take more conscious responsibility for it? Van Manen, drawing on Turner, indicates how such practice is nevertheless a certain kind of activity that can be cultivated:

> . . . in spite of this intangibility, the concept of practice must include the connotation of something transferable, teachable, transmittable, or reproducible.
>
> (Van Manen, 1999b)

Van Manen is writing here about the practice of teaching. However, for the purposes of this chapter, we wish to consider practice in relation to the question of whether the integrative scholarly development (in terms of head, heart and hand) can be actively cultivated, and in what sense an opening to the creativity of unspecialisation can be practised.

This direction has been pursued by several writers under different rubrics, in different contexts. This includes Bachelard's (1964/2004) notion of 'reverie', Gadamer's (1975/1997) concept of 'play' and mytho-poetic directions for education (MacDonald, 1981; Willis, 2005). In particular, Heidegger (1959/1966), in his writings on contemplative thinking, gives us some helpful directions about the sense in which such an opening to *being* can be 'practised'. His argument is associated with a long-standing tradition of what Keats has called 'negative capability' (see, for example, Claxton, 1997, for a fuller discussion of this logic). Negative capability means the natural 'generativity' that arises, not by positively seeking integration in a goal-directed way, but by allowing integration 'to be'. This occurs during periods of 'letting go', 'lying fallow' or having space and time for what has been called 'blue skies thinking'. (See, for example, Claxton, 1997, for fuller discussion of this logic.)

In an essay entitled 'The Age of the World Picture', Heidegger (1977) cautioned against the tendency to secure the precedence of 'methodology' over 'presence' as a way of 'opening to understanding'. He was concerned that the way science was being organised and practised resulted in the 'scholar' disappearing and the 'research worker' becoming a technologist whose specialising concerns prematurely closes down the creativity of unspecialisation in a self-referenced and self-reifying way:

> The human becomes that being upon which all that is, is grounded as regards the manner of its Being and its truth. The human becomes the relational centre of that which is as such.
>
> (Heidegger, 1977, p. 128; translation adapted from the original German)

Such a self-referencing, specialised perspective forms the foundation of what Heidegger called calculative thinking. It is characterised by a thinking that is preoccupied with existing patterns in the way we organise, categorise and particularise phenomena.

Heidegger distinguished contemplative thinking from calculative thinking. Our argument proposes that it is contemplative thinking that is centrally relevant to the question of whether the creativity of unspecialisation can be practised. Contemplative thinking is about how one can think in a receptive way that is open to the excess of being beyond oneself (being-in-the-world) and not the more calculative type of thinking that is 'always on the move' and merely 'doing' an existing pattern of organised thought.

This does not mean that such presence and openness to 'being-in-the-world' is passive. There *is* a certain 'waiting' in it; but that waiting is a form of actively practising a 'negative capability' that keeps at bay the kind of possessive 'willing' that prematurely grasps at what is already known. In this way, contemplative thinking can be said to be actively practised in the sense that it holds open the willingness of not knowing, and so allows a release into the openness and creativity of a more unspecialised realm: "We must develop the art of waiting, releasing our hold . . ." (Hixon, 1989, p. 4). And this is not far away. It is very near; nearer than our habitual ways of thinking. In releasing ourselves from our more habitual thinking, a less specialised presence is possible, one that is open to profiles of the world that are at the edge of the known, where novelty occurs.

> Openness is not due to any specific point of view but is rather the absence of single-perspective perceiving and thinking.
>
> (Hixon, 1989, p. 9).

In relation to an integrative vision of scholarship, we thus wish to include the creativity of unspecialisation. Heidegger has provided us with clues for a more contemplative direction in this pursuit; one that is receptive, but that can nevertheless be practised by actively becoming aware of an alternative to calculative thinking. But we would like to take this one step further and propose some directions for such practice based on Eugene Gendlin's philosophy of 'entry into the implicit' (Gendlin, 1991). Gendlin's notion of 'the implicit' refers to the place where unspecialised possibilities have their life. Entry into the implicit then involves an experiential movement that allows the aliveness of the implicit to be sensed and to function as an ongoing creative source of possible new meanings. As such, Gendlin provides one possible practice that can serve scholarly integration through the remembrance to discipline our specialised concerns and thus give way to the 'letting be' our more unspecialised possibilities.

In his philosophy of entry into the implicit, Gendlin sets out a relational ontology in which contemplative thinking can be practised by attending to one's own lived body and, as such, opens up the excesses of being-in-the-world beyond pre-existing patterns.

Gendlin's philosophy as a practice of opening the creativity of unspecialisation

Gendlin's philosophy of entry into the implicit (Gendlin, 1991) builds on the thoughts of Heidegger and Merleau-Ponty. It focuses on how the lived body can open profiles of the world beyond pre-patterned thought. The phrase 'entry into the implicit' means that words, thoughts and representations are formulated and come from an experiential practice based on attending to the lived body's sense of felt meaning in any moment. Two practices arise out of this philosophy. One is called 'focusing', the other, 'thinking at the edge'.

Focusing

Focusing describes an experiential practice of attending to the relationship between language and the aliveness or excess of what language is trying to point to, by grounding such aliveness in the lived body's *felt* sense. Through a felt sense, meaning is apprehended in a holistic way that is more than its formulation in language and already-patterned thought. The felt sense is full of the excess of the life-world – its fleshly textures and abundances of meanings. The felt-sense is ". . . implicitly intricate in a way that is more than what is already formed or distinguished" (Gendlin, 1992, p. 347). The practice of focusing is then a body-based hermeneutics that goes back and forth between this 'more than' of the lifeworld and the many ways of patterning the lifeworld, as it comes to form in language and thought.

Thinking at the edge

Thinking at the edge is a stepped process that uses focusing but builds theory from the freshness of the focusing process. In such a way, it aims ". . . to think and speak about our world and our selves by generating terms from a felt sense. Such terms formulate experiential intricacy rather than turning everything we think about into externally viewed objects" (Gendlin, 2004a).

Opening up unspecialised possibilities

Both these practices may provide direction for how to open unspecialised possibilities through an embodied contemplative approach. In order to illustrate this in a concrete way, let us refer to an illustration that Gendlin provides (the use of ellipses [. . .] in the following passage refers to the 'more than words can say' of the felt sense:

> An artist stands before an unfinished picture, pondering it, seeing, feeling, bodily sensing it, having a . . . Suppose the artist's . . . is one of some dissatisfaction. Is that an emotional reaction, simply a feeling-tone? No

indeed. Implicit in the . . . is the artist's training, experience with many designs, and much else. But more: the . . . is also the implying of the next line, which has not yet come. The artist ponders 'what it needs'. It needs some line, some erasure, something moved over, something . . . The artist tries this and that, and something else, and erases it again each time. The . . . is quite demanding. It recognizes the failure of each attempt. It seems to know precisely what it wants and it knows that those attempts are not it. Rather than accepting those, a good artist prefers to leave a design unfinished, sometimes for years.

(Gendlin, 1992, p. 348)

This illustration shows how the lived body is an important gate to the alive and implicit 'more' where unspecialised possibilities can be touched. So, in answer to our earlier question of whether unspecialisation can be practised, we suggest that it can, and that Gendlin offers important understandings and practices that, although active in a certain sense, can honour the kind of contemplative attitude that is hospitable to being addressed by new meanings from 'the more' as we pursue scholarly enquiry.

In relation to contemplative scholarly practice relevant to care, we can imagine the following vignette. Sarah, a nurse, has been struggling on the ward with a deep sense of discomfort she experienced in a case conference. This discomfort is highly complex but implicitly 'there' in the 'more' of her felt sense. 'In it' is the 'head', 'hand' and 'heart' as already together. But as she settles and lets go of her specialised concern to be a competent staff nurse and even her specialised concern to be professional, scholarly and caring, she attends to what wants to come from her felt sense of the whole of everything together there. Her discomfort carries a number of different dimensions: how she had recently read a scholarly work on Levinas that led her to think about the nature of respect, how certain experiences in her past professional and personal life had impressed upon her the importance of being careful not to assume what another needs, and how all this and some other things gave her a sense of possible directions of action that were consistent with the uncomfortable feeling of what was missing in terms of the kind of respectful care that she would like to offer in this particular situation. In this situation she thus actively made space for a more contemplative approach to the integration of head , hand and heart that was implicit in the 'pre-formed' unspecialisation of her felt sense. Yet this was productive. A clear understanding and possible action did come, that was ultimately supported in a way that included what could be called an integrated way of being as articulated in this chapter.

Conclusion

We have tried to set out the idea of a more contemplative scholarship, one that draws on a natural movement in 'being' to embody and live in a knowing, valuing and action-oriented way. We looked at historical evidence before the 'doing' of integration became such a dilemma and highlighted a virtue that is inherent in our unspecialised possibilities of being, while at the same time questioning how our specialised engagements can be held more vitally within these unspecialised movements. In particular, in relation to scholarship for caring practices, we noted how empathic imagination is a central faculty for integrating the head, hand and heart.

So why are contemplative practices important for the kind of scholarship that acknowledges an integration of head, hand and heart? In an increasingly specialised and even fragmented world, the humming integration of head, hand and heart that naturally occurs becomes easily obscured by the excessive compartmentalisation of attention to specialised tasks. The essence of creativity requires the kind of space that only comes with a slowing down, an in-breath, that for a moment releases a relentless hold. The kind of integrative focus offered in this chapter may thus suggest some interesting directions for consideration as to how contemplative orientations for practice can be supported, guarded and nurtured.

10 Complex knowledge to underpin caring
Embodied relational understanding

In the last chapter we considered the need for a more complex epistemology and scholarship that could provide a foundation for humanly sensitive care. Within this spirit we discussed *phronesis* (actionable knowledge), empathy, and the challenge of integrating science, art and morality as touchstones for the kind of more holistic knowing that we believe humanly sensitive care needs. In this present chapter, we deepen some of these epistemological considerations with specific reference to nursing practice and name 'embodied relational understanding' as the kind of knowing that is complex enough to underpin caring. Further, in acknowledging the underrepresented aesthetic dimension of knowing, we begin to explore the possibilities of more aesthetic research-based descriptions that can expand existing preconceptions of what is called 'evidence based practice'.

We are particularly interested in the kinds of knowledge and evidence that can provide direction for a more humanly sensitive care. This concern has led us as qualitative researchers to consider how best to engage readers with research findings in ways that have the potential to meaningfully impact on practice and education.

This concern has engaged us in thinking further about two interrelated issues: the kind of knowledge that is particularly relevant to caring practices and the way in which qualitative research findings can serve such knowledge. Inclusion of latter issues occurs not because we wish to exclude other forms of knowledge and enquiry, but because, as qualitative researchers we have wished to refine the contribution that a particular kind of phenomenological research can make to caring practices. With this in mind the chapter progresses as follows:

1. A consideration of knowledge for caring practices: embodied relational understanding.
2. The value of transforming phenomenological research findings: towards a more aesthetic phenomenology.
3. An outline of embodied interpretation: evidence for the head, hand and heart.

4.   Understanding the experience of stroke: an application of embodied interpretation.

A consideration of knowledge for caring: Embodied relational understanding

It has long been acknowledged that the various kinds and levels of knowledge that are relevant to caring practices are much more complex than our traditional notion of propositional knowledge (Benner, 1984, 1994; Boyer, 1990; Carper, 1978; Riley, Beal, Levi & McCausland, 2002; Schon, 1983; Van Manen, 1994, 1999a, and others). There is also a body of knowledge that addresses the complex ways by which professionals make judgements and decisions in practice, ranging from the intuitive (Benner, 1984; Polkinghorne, 2004) to the analytical (Buckingham & Adams, 2000a, 2000b). As previously discussed, knowledge for caring practices does not easily break down into traditional disciplinary categories such as science, arts and ethics.

In both the modernist and postmodernist eras, there have been various attempts to articulate the kind of knowledge that is inclusive of the 'head', 'hand' and 'heart' (objective truth, actionable knowledge and empathic knowledge). This more complex view of knowledge is relevant to nursing (and any caring profession) because immersion in practice demands a way to overcome the 'deep inseparability' of truth, ethics and action in the complex and marginal situations that nurses have to manage. So within this discourse we have been interested in the question: what kinds of knowledge can guide practice in complex human situations? And we have developed our own characterisation of the kind of knowledge that can encompass knowledge for the head, hand and heart which we call 'embodied relational under-standing' (Todres, 2008).

Embodied relational understanding refers to a way of knowing that is holistically contextual; that is, a form of knowledge that is attentive to the rich and moving flow of individuals lives in relation to others, is attentive to very specific situations and to the inner worlds of what it is like for patients to 'go through something'. This kind of knowing includes the resource of technical evidence and propositional knowledge (what we have metaphorised as the 'head'), but integrates this with the specificity of 'just this' practical situation (what we have metaphorised as the 'hand'), as well as an imaginative-ethical capacity of the inner world of the patient (what we have metaphorised as the 'heart'). When these three sensibilities are integrated the result may be said to be 'holistic', in that it is inclusive of these three domains of knowledge. Furthermore, such knowledge may be considered to re-present what Gendlin (1974) referred to as 'a thick pattern' of knowing, in which the holistic 'weave' of living relationships (the lifeworld) is a complex and inclusive resource for guiding knowledge. Therefore, as a knowledge resource, the 'thickness of living' points to the rich and moving flow of the contextual world as it is humanly lived (including its 'insides'), and we would wish that any understanding that is relevant to caring be informed by such complex knowing; a complex knowing that is aesthetically textured and sensitive to unique situations. We refer to this kind of inclusive contextual, holistic, and aesthetically textured knowledge as embodied relational understanding.

In any given practice situation there is something unique and novel; it is never simply a duplication of a previous situation – it is live and ongoing. Thus 'the known' is always meeting 'the unknown' and the term 'relational' is a particular challenge for knowledge; that is, that the application of any knowledge is always in relation to a specific concrete occurrence that can never be fully encompassed from previous knowledge. But more than this there can be no knowledge in a practice situation without an embodied practitioner there. In referring to the notion of 'an embodiment of knowledge' we are indicating something that is quite complex and has within it a practitioner that embodies knowledge, but also much more than knowledge: in their engagement, practitioners are 'a locus of intersection' of specialised knowledge, of historical, personal and professional experience and – in the applied mood – of a willingness to look freshly at what this unknown situation needs. Holding on too tightly to knowledge here, needing too much certainty, reduces the range of possible applied resources that are adequate to an actionable epistemology where 'thick' knowledge is required. By sharing worlds, human beings can know in participative ways, and this opens up the possibility of empathy, in addition to specialised knowledge. Embodied relational understanding brings all these considerations together and indicates an empathic understanding of another's world, drawing on resources of both knowing and openness, and applying these resources relationally in very specific and concrete circumstances.

So why is embodied relational understanding particularly important as a foundation for humanly sensitive care? For a number of reasons: it provides a complex enough epistemology that can give 'heart' and empathy to caring practices; it is an involved form of knowing that brings 'the self' into play, drawing on complex thoughtful resources of the nurse; and it includes an openness to the 'unique and alive otherness' of the situation or patient's needs, which call for the empathic imagination.

There are all kinds of ways that embodied relational understanding can be facilitated. For example there is a rich tradition of reflective practice that is germane to this goal (Ekebergh, 2007; Finlay, 2002, 2008; Finlay & Gough, 2003). In the field of personal and professional development there are disciplines and practices that increase empathic imagination and ethical sensitivity (Biley & Champney-Smith, 2003; Harrison, 2006; Hunter, 2002; Madden, 1990; Schuster, 1994; Stowe, 1996; Weems, 2009; Willis, 2005). In addition there is a strong tradition of philosophical and literary topics that have been pursued within health-related humanities as a complement to biomedical science (Carel, 2008; Evans, Ahlzen, Heath & Mcnaughton, 2008). In this chapter however we would like to consider how phenomenological research findings have a particularly powerful role to play in facilitating embodied relational understanding in readers and audiences and thus empower the possibility of more humanly sensitive care. It is not that we are suggesting that phenomenological research findings are the only way to empower humanly sensitive care; rather we wish to indicate how a novel way of transforming phenomenological findings can offer one interesting direction for serving embodied relational understanding.

The value of transforming phenomenological research findings: Towards a more aesthetic phenomenology

What kind of research evidence can provide direction for a more humanly sensitive care? In our view, just as there may be strengths that quantitative research contributes to embodied relational understanding, there are characteristics of qualitative research that are particularly conducive to facilitating embodied relational understanding in readers. Qualitative research accesses the complexity of peoples' everyday experiences in an open-ended, discovery-oriented way, and within a richly detailed context. When well communicated, it capitalises on the insider perspective of the lifeworld to evocatively portray what particular experiences and events are like for the people living through them. However, the way that qualitative research findings are often presented is not necessarily sufficient to communicate the thick knowledge that embodied relational understanding would ask for (Halling, 2002). The concern to sensitise practice may benefit from an approach that transforms rigorous qualitative research findings into more evocative re-presentations. Such a translational approach attends to the scientific concern of utilising rigorously derived research findings, and in a further step, attends more closely to the communicative concern of re-presenting these findings in more evocative and humanly sensitive ways (Todres & Holloway, 2004). The kind of transformation that we are aiming for is one that can produce knowledge for the 'head', 'hand' and 'heart'. There is a body of work within the nursing literature that describes how poetry and other forms of evocative re-presentations of people's experience and/or qualitative research findings have been used in both practice and the education of nurses (Birx, 1994; Chan, 2003a; Harrison, 2006; Hunter, 2002; Öhlen, 2003; Raingruber, 2009; Triestman, 1986). We have taken this concern towards the direction of a more aesthetic form of phenomenology.

So what do we mean by a more *aesthetic* phenomenology? Phenomenology based on Husserl's project aims to clarify phenomena by succinctly describing their quidity (the 'whatness' of a phenomenon , its essential boundaries or 'bare bones'). It thus concentrates on a concern to elucidate the structure of phenomena, the invariant properties that cohere through variant individual cases. A more aesthetic phenomenology is much more concerned with texture rather than structure (Todres, 1998), that is, a concern to portray the lived 'sensuous taste' of what an experience may be and feel like. Whereas an emphasis on structure tends to employ language in its most summative forms, a concern to evoke texture employs a poetic sensibility to point to the felt dimensions of experience. Language within this context can thus be understood as providing a kind of 'experiential direction' rather than an 'analytical summation'. Husserlian descriptive phenomenology aims for analytical summation and thus may use language that, without care, has the potential to kill a sense of the 'aliveness' of experiential phenomena, by necessarily emphasising its more abstract essence. A more aesthetic phenomenology is less concerned with such summations and rather emphasises the textures of experience by using directional or 'pointing' language that evokes the experience (Willis, 2004). A further implication of the concern to communicate texture in research findings, is that such portrayals may have the potential to transform the reader or audience in ways that good poetry does, in that it can move or touch us. Such 'evidence' thus takes on an emotionally impactful timbre and thus can be very conducive to the kind of personal and professional development that stretches the empathic imagination and, as such, supports the cultivation of ethical sensitivity. In this way a more aesthetic phenomenology is a highly conducive route to embodied relational understanding.

In pursuing a more aesthetic phenomenology we have developed an approach for transforming phenomenological research findings that we call 'embodied interpretation', and which we develop further in the next chapter. The goal of embodied interpretation shares a value with poetry to evocatively facilitate a kind of 'emotional homecoming', a kind of existential recognition of experiential phenomena in which one can find the 'I' in the 'Thou' in Buber's (1970) sense, and which forges a human connection between the reader and the phenomena that is descriptively portrayed; forging a bond between the personal and the interpersonal. It is the aesthetic quality of language that makes words carry a human bond, this means that words are not just technical. Therefore, we are interested in finding words that can be faithful to the experience being shown in all its rich detail, complexity and texture, and which can make a space for such a bond. Such words can open up an intersubjective space, give freedom to readers to make a personal connection with the phenomenon, and enable readers to experience a resonance with the written description (Hirschfield, 1998). Such words are experienced as 'how they feel'. And it is this 'how they feel' that guided us in looking for a process that connected language to its embodied 'feel'. Gendlin's philosophy of the implicit has helped us in this pursuit, particularly his focus on the vibrant tension between words and the bodily felt sense of 'more than words can say'. As such, Gendlin shows how the epistemic body (the body that senses and knows) is a crucial faculty for holistic knowing: the bodily felt sense gives textured meaning to words, even though these bodily textured meanings are in excess of the words. We have used many of Gendlin's insights, as elaborated in the next chapter when developing the process of embodied interpretation. But here, we would like to illustrate how we have used this process of embodied interpretation to re-present the findings of lifeworld-oriented research in more evocative ways. As such we show how one possible aesthetically informed methodology can serve to facilitate embodied relational understanding in readers.

Understanding the experience of stroke: Three illustrations of embodied interpretation

For the present chapter we draw upon three published phenomenological research studies, which describe experiences of adjusting to life after suffering a stroke. Using a 'berry-picking' method (Bates, 1989) we specifically chose papers that provided enough rich description of the studies' findings that would facilitate an embodied interpretative process. Here we found Cash's (2009) criteria useful when choosing research findings. These include: substantive contribution, aesthetic merit, reflexivity, impact and expression of reality. All three studies were phenomenological accounts of living after stroke (Hjelmblink, Bernsten, Uvhagen, Kunkel & Holstrom, 2007; Kvigne & Kirkevold, 2003; Murray & Harrison, 2004). As the purpose here is to illustrate the potential of embodied interpretation to increase shared understanding, we only use certain aspects of these findings to show some evocative possibilities that emerge. We thus cannot do justice to the full complexity of the phenomena explored in each paper and encourage readers to seek out the original papers. We now present three embodied inter-pretations, one from each study, in each case focusing on an aspect of the experience of living with stroke that was derived from each paper.

1) Embodied Interpretation from Kvigne and Kirkevold (2003), 'Living with bodily strangeness: Women's experiences of their changing and unpredictable body following stroke'.

Betrayed

Strong as a bear
never sick, me
I carried on through it all
a woman's steel
maybe
so strong, held the weight
of everyone
on me
never paid much attention to you,
taken for granted body

over those days, hours
you became a stranger
you were not *me*

my dependable friend, my 'do it all' body,
something was wrong
the doctor couldn't see inside
but I could feel you strangely
changed.
I awoke to an unreal body
There
laid cold on the floor alone.

This hand, couldn't finish that letter
Refused
I walked
you forgot
you brought me down
Refused
Foot, listen
Arm, please heed
I *will* you
painstaking
I have tried to slowly instruct you
agonisingly direct you
but you knock over the flowers, smash crockery, topple the table
forget the right words, names
piss over me
betrayer
you are unruly and slow,
too slow
Demander
let down, I am shamed.

2) Embodied Interpretation from Murray and Harrison (2004), 'The meaning and experience of being a stroke survivor: An interpretative phenomenological analysis'. The aspect that we have focused on is 'the invisibility of emotional difficulties'.

Invisible

Look at me
I look alright
people wouldn't know
Don't understand, there is
A problem.

Look at him
he would say there is nothing wrong with me
I wish I had a broken leg

people could relate to a broken leg
They don't understand
why I cry sometimes
for nothing
I cry sometimes
for nothing
Anything can set it off
Anything.

People wonder what is wrong with me
I grin when I shouldn't
I laugh when I shouldn't
I cry when I shouldn't
Anything can set it off

They can't see
what is really happening
unexpected noise
makes me angry
Anything can set it off

I wish my emotional disability
could be seen
people could relate
they would understand
why I grin, laugh, cry
when I shouldn't
why I am angry.

3) Hjelmblink et al. (2007), 'Understanding the meaning of rehabilitation to an aphasic patient through phenomenological analysis – a case study'. The aspect that we have focused on is the experience of aphasia and the lost expression of oneself as a thinking and acting person.

Words cut out

Since the Stroke
left side of head
I am different from them
they melt their words
I have shards to share
cut off thoughts can't move between, can they?
I live behind a broken screen
I am on the outside of life now
I have to adapt, but this destroys my chance of talking success
I hear them . . . life's conversations

coarsing words pour out
rippling against the sides and flowing out into life sea
water inter-courses, over-lapping worlds
My word spring spits
clatters river rocks and pebbles,
splits stones.
Stuff of dams and rubble stilts transactions
scrambles up bits, scree, flint, then . . .
when no word comes
grit forces
to complete the transaction.
Unnatural encounters in an alien language
Are bits a thinking person?
Splinters of reality, cut ups of who I am, of where I have been, bits of
    what is
and is not
Did they receive . . . a mistake?
cut off, I drift
live on the inside now
I absorb the room's silent shame,
or check what was said
I hold back to make natural encounters
with an alien language more comfortable for them.

Discussion

In this final section we would like to consider the value of these research-
based translations for enhancing the kind of empathic understanding that
may be needed for a more humanly sensitive care. In what ways may the three
embodied interpretations offered above support the kind of knowledge that
communicates both the heart and the head of the matter?

In the final analysis it is only readers or audiences of embodied interpretations that can say how these interpretations 'spoke to them', engaged
them in heartfelt ways, and also led them to a deeper understanding of the
nature of the experience. We would like to consider, however, why it is
entirely plausible that the aesthetics of the embodied interpretations offered
work to facilitate the kind of embodied relational understanding that is
particularly important for humanly sensitive care . In the first embodied
interpretation, the text circles around the felt dilemma of feeling betrayed by
'her' body in nuanced and intense ways. In the second embodied interpretation, the text circles around the felt dilemma of having become an
outsider, misunderstood by others who cannot see 'her' disability and cannot
understand the source of her emotional reactions. In the third embodied
interpretation the text circles around the felt dilemma of being hindered from
expressing 'himself' in taken-for-granted ways.

In our view, the added value of re-presenting findings through embodied interpretation concerns two particular strengths that are central to a poetic language that is grounded in bodily feeling: wholeness and existentiality (Hirschfield, 1998). Poetic language emphasises 'wholeness' in that, through rhythm, repetition, and imagery, a wholeness is pointed to that is more than what is there. Such poetic showing points to an implicit wholeness which asks readers to stretch themselves and to participate in imaginative and personal ways. Poetic language emphasises a concern with existentiality in that it refers to the impact of our concrete human existence: 'this pain', happening to 'this unique' person.

Such concrete occurrence is very specific but paradoxically has the power to touch our common humanity. Such existentiality is achieved by poetic writing that goes back and forth between what is happening to this unique experiencing person and the indications and whispers of its more general existential significance. This play between the particular and general may offer a certain poignancy or intensity by which a human experience can be shown as both unique and shared.

Conclusion: A kind of knowledge for supporting humanly sensitive care

In conclusion we would like to indicate two ways in which re-presentations of research findings through embodied interpretation may be fruitfully used: as an expanded form of evidence for nursing practice and, as an educational resource for facilitating empathic understanding.

An expanded form of evidence

We believe that in any caring context, judgements about what to do are informed not just by conventional notions of evidence (propositional and technical knowledge) but also by the complexity of living caring situations. This calls for human-relevant understandings that are not best accessed through formal sources but rather through the ability to make a human connection with what is encountered (Polkinghorne, 2004; Todres, 2008). It is within this aspiration towards expanded forms of evidence that embodied interpretation, as a novel way of re-presenting qualitative research, may have a valuable role to play. We can imagine professional carers availing themselves of embodied interpretations that have been undertaken with a range of health and illness experiences. These may be useful in such circumstances, as an additional resource where judgements require a more holistic and 'inner-world' appreciation of the person's needs and requirements for care.

An educational resource for facilitating empathic understanding

We believe that embodied interpretations of health and illness experiences can be fruitfully used by educators when the aim is to sensitise health and social care students in a way that offers experiential directions rather than mere summative descriptions of the human dimensions of the experience. The task to 'sensitise' is not best achieved by including more information, but rather by the more 'aesthetic-holistic' challenge to make a phenomenon more palpably present. This embodied emphasis that draws on one's own bodily awareness enriches 'experiential knowing' in that it provides a kind of knowing that is full of personal meaning that is deeply felt. Educational methodologies that facilitate 'palpable presence' offer a connection to the experience of the other and can act as a resource in their professional lives. We can imagine how a range of educational approaches can engage students in more embodied and poetic forms of understanding through the use of embodied interpretations. In our view such an educational strategy is one way to orient learners to the more human dimensions of care.

Although there is an interesting groundswell of alternative approaches for offering expanded forms of evidence (Benner & Chesla, 1998; Polkinghorne, 2004), as well as alternative educational resources for facilitating empathic understanding (Chan, 2003b, 2010; Darbyshire, 1994; Davis & Schafer, 1995; Harrison, 2006; Raingruber, 2009), the present chapter offers a distinctive approach towards these aspirations that begin from a research-base grounded in research participants' experiences, rather than an approach that is based on reflective resources of practitioners and their clinical experience alone. Embodied interpretation as a way of re-presenting qualitative research findings thus offers a knowledge base that wishes to honour both the value of research as well as the personal resources of practitioners when acting in complex caring situations.

11 Embodied interpretation
One way of re-presenting research findings that may serve to sensitise the empathic imagination

In this third part of the book, 'Developing the capacity to care', we have been exploring the possibility of an epistemology that we believe is particularly conducive to the phenomenon of caring. With reference to the metaphors of 'the head' and 'the heart', we have considered the kind of knowledge that is needed to *understand* care, and the ways in which knowledge needs to be communicated in order to evoke and sensitise the *capacity* for care. This chapter provides one illustration of an approach for the communication of caring-related phenomena that may serve to deepen the empathic feeling capacities of readers and professionals. Building on Chapter 10 we will unfold in greater detail some of the methodological nuances in this approach, as well as its epistemological foundation.

As qualitative researchers our work has involved a striving to articulate the significant experiences of others in health and social contexts, where peoples' meaningful experiences get lost in systems and technology. Increasingly, our attempts to understand such human experiences and to communicate their significance to readers have changed our practice of phenomenology, especially in the way we engage in the hermeneutic process and how we re-present our findings. We call this process 'embodied interpretation'. It builds upon an intense curiosity around the aesthetic dimensions of phenomenology, a tradition that goes back to Heidegger's interest in poetry (Heidegger, 1971) and Gadamer's writings on the relevance of the beautiful (Gadamer, 1986).

Embodied interpretation is different from traditional descriptive phenomenology in the Husserlian sense, which uses language in rigorous, precise and rational ways to show the boundaries of experienced phenomena. There is a tendency within this more traditional concern to use language in summative ways that can oversterilise or even deaden the aliveness of the shown phenomena. Within this emphasis, significant meanings can become imprisoned within a scientific notion of essences. The particular challenge is to find words that are faithful to the phenomenon in all its complexity, sense and texture. A more aesthetic phenomenology therefore uses language in more evocative and poetic ways.

In this chapter we wish to show a process where we listen to what people say in order to *carry forward* the meanings that these words open up. We also indicate our epistemological stance, which legitimises re-wording what individual people say in such a way that it may enliven intersubjective understanding and insight about phenomena that have both shared and unique dimensions. But first we wish to say something about a more aesthetic direction for phenomenology.

The direction and value of a more aesthetic phenomenology

A more aesthetic phenomenology shares its values with poetry: to evocatively facilitate a particular kind of emotional 'homecoming'. We use the term 'emotional homecoming' as a metaphor for the emotional recognition of a truth that is also deeply personal, familiar, meaningful and authentic. Such an experience of homecoming has within it a deep feeling of recognition that may be characterised by the kind of ontological weight that connects us to the place where we feel both deeply ourselves as well as deeply connected to our common humanity. We are aware that our reference to the term 'common humanity' is a perspective not shared by all social scientists. We would like to acknowledge that there is an ongoing debate in both philosophy and social science and that the extremes of this debate either emphasise uniqueness or commonality. However an existential phenomenological perspective that is consistent with the spirit of this chapter does not take either of these extremes, and we will elaborate on this in the next section that outlines our episte- mological framework. Suffice it to say for now that there are dimensions of the human experience that may touch on certain common human structures. For example Heidegger (1927/1962) provides one way of articulating funda- mental shared dimensions as 'existentials', which include temporality; spatiality and embodiment. He helpfully differentiates between the 'onto- logical', which speaks of the existential preconditions of being human and the 'ontic', in which there are many uniquely different individual and cultural ways of experiencing such ontological structures.

Within a more aesthetic phenomenology, words are not just tools or skills that are performed; they are also experienced for how they *feel*, and this 'how they feel' – the inner dimension of language – is an aesthetic quality that is central to the process of understanding. Feeling a word does not necessarily make it aesthetically more valuable than a word that we do not feel. We are not claiming that the feel of language is all that there is to understanding – just that in poetic discourse it achieves particular attention. Such language that locates us in relation to others is both personal and interpersonal. When the feel of language is operating, we are in touch with its aesthetic qualities and sense of fit. This aesthetic quality of language is the thing that makes words human and much more than just technical.

We would like to emphasise that words which connect the personal to the interpersonal world are humanising in that they can find the 'I' in the 'Thou' in Buber's sense (Buber, 1970). This is assisted by the kind of language that is evocative and poetic and that seeks to make things come alive. We seek to find a way of using language so that readers of phenomenological descriptions can find personal meaning in the descriptions, and thus find themselves *in* the language in some way. Language can then connect to people in a heartfelt way and be complex enough to awaken not just a logical understanding but the sense of it as it lives. This lived experience is in excess of the words; it is more than words can say.

Van Manen (1999a, 2006) has written about what it takes for a text to 'speak' to us, or to 'call' and 'stir' us, and recommends qualities that can be acknowledged in the way we use language to serve these purposes. They include:

- How descriptions, through being concrete, can bring nearness or presence to the phenomena they are referring to.
- How to indicate something of the phenomenon as a whole movement.
- How to intensify certain meanings through repetition, alliteration and other poetic devices.
- How to allow readers or an audience to relate to and resonate with the shown phenomenon in unique ways.
- How to show the ethical 'call' from the 'other' and how this can be invoked both in style and content.

In the following quote Seamus Heaney indicates the power of poetic representation to facilitate an experience of emotional 'homecoming':

> Poetic form is both the ship and the anchor. It is at once a buoyancy and a holding, allowing for the simultaneous gratification of whatever is centrifugal and centripetal in mind and body. And it is by such means that Yeats's work does what the necessary poetry always does, which is to touch the base of our sympathetic nature while taking in at the same time the unsympathetic reality of the world to which that nature is constantly exposed. The form of the poem, in other words, is crucial to poetry's power to do the thing which always is and always will be to poetry's credit: the power to persuade that vulnerable part of our consciousness of its rightness in spite of the evidence of wrongness all around it.
>
> (Heaney, 1995, pp. 466–467)

The experience of emotional homecoming is particularly important in the health and social care context, as illness and vulnerability have been essentially characterised as an experience of not feeling at home in the world or in one's body (Toombs, 2002).

As qualitative researchers, we attempt to facilitate the experience of emotional homecoming by acting as evocative mediators who add ontological weight to common existential issues. We are aware that the role of 'evocative mediator' may be considered controversial. With regard to the expression 'evocative', our view is that all writing is evocative to some degree. With regard to the role of 'mediator', rather than wishing to prescribe meanings, as mediators, we wish to be more open-ended by indicating the *freedom for personal resonance* given to audiences when one uses more poetic language. We are arguing that there is more meaning in a language that is expressed in this way than in a language that is overly defined and summative. It could paradoxically be argued that language that is too definitive in its conclusions is limiting. Thus as evocative mediators we attempt to offer words that can open up the 'between' of intersubjective space.

Epistemological framework

Before we describe the nature of 'embodied interpretation' and its potential application as a novel way of evocatively re-presenting meanings in phenomenological research, we wish to situate our approach within an interpretive epistemology that acknowledges the evocative power of language to *carry forward* meanings that are neither only unique nor only shared, but always 'in between'. Such an epistemology may support a poetically informed aesthetic phenomenology which re-presents others' words in different ways. Thus we would like to briefly indicate this epistemology which draws primarily on the work of Gadamer (1975/1997) and Gendlin (2004b):

> Phenomenology has no problem going beyond a single person's private experiencing because experiencing is inherently an interaction process in a situation with other people and things. What appears is neither internal nor external, neither just private nor just interactional. My situation is not just 'subjective' since the others in it are more than I can experience, but neither is it 'objective' since my situation does not exist apart from me.
>
> (Gendlin, 2004b, pp. 147–148)

In aesthetic phenomenology we seek words to bring human experiences 'to life' so that they can be understood between us and amongst us. Whose experience is then understood? After Gadamer, we would have to say that the experience that one understands is neither fully one's own, nor is it another's alone. We thus do not understand something in the same way as another person (as in an objectivist view of the world, where words would correspond exactly to something described). Nor do we understand something completely uniquely and personally (as in a subjectivist view of the world where words only have private meaning). Within an aesthetically informed, phenomenologically based research into others' experiences, we do not believe that we have to stick to the same words as an informant in order to illuminate an experience like homelessness or pain. Yes, we attend very closely to the experiential world that the informant's word-expressions open up, the horizons and lively evocative happenings that the words signify. But, we also stand before such a world as an instance of something that has shareable dimensions within a meaningful world-with-others. To understand is then to understand both something of this unique individual and the shared intersubjective horizons within which any unique experience occurs.

So far, so Gadamer.

But we also do not stick to the same words as an informant for another reason, which in our view is best articulated by Gendlin's body-based hermeneutics. Such an approach emphasises an understanding 'with-the-body' that includes aesthetic texture as one of its inclusive dimensions. This is an understanding with both 'head' and 'heart' (see Todres, 2007, for a more extensive elaboration of such embodied enquiry).

Within this perspective, Gendlin's body-based hermeneutics results in an approach that engages researchers with the question of 'what we found in our bodily sensed understanding when listening to others' meanings and experiences'. Such bodily sensed understanding is an event where meaning 'comes home' to persons. To offer this possibility to readers in their own way may perhaps best be communicated by researchers who have made a temporary experiential and personal 'home' for the understanding themselves. Such understanding carries a 'fresh' dimension, but not from nowhere. It is in this context that we substantially draw upon Gendlin's notion of the 'carrying forward' of bodily alive meanings as an important contribution to interpretive phenomenology. We are aware that Gendlin is best known within the psychotherapy arena and that the relevance of Gendlin's work to qualitative research methodology may not be widely known or understood. However, it should be remembered that Gendlin was a philosopher before he was a psychotherapist and that early work focused on epistemological issues. (See for example, his paper on 'experiential phenomenology'; Gendlin, 1973.) He has returned to some of these epistemological issues more recently (see for example, Gendlin, 2004b, on 'carrying forward'). He has applied his experiential phenomenology, not just for therapeutic purposes, but also within the context of a wider approach to research and enquiry, an approach he calls 'thinking at the edge' (Krycka, 2006). The present chapter builds on this foundation. However within the constraints of this chapter we are unable revisit all of the debates about Gendlin's relevance for qualitative research and refer readers to Todres (1999, 2004b, 2007).

We do not just wish to restate Gendlin's work but rather wish to show a novel application of 'carrying forward' by means of embodied interpretation. However, we do need to revisit some of Gendlin's key ideas on this topic as a framework for our own approach.

The idea of 'carrying forward' can be understood with reference to Gendlin's (2004b, p. 133) assertion that ". . . we have much more than the concepts – we have language forming freshly and oddly to say all this. And we have what language can freshly speak from, which is anything but indeterminate".

Gendlin calls such understanding – that has both a fresh aliveness that functions, as well as a grounded history that has gone before it – 'carrying forward'. It is an understanding that has something old and something new. How else can understanding be relevant if it does not carry new implications and thus live freshly for people in new situations and contexts?

The term 'carrying forward' can be seen to indicate an aesthetically inclusive form of understanding and conforms to the following characteristics (this characterisation is a modification of Gendlin, 2004b):

- It starts in openness to 'otherness' in that it can be informed by others' experiences and meanings. It begins at this 'juncture'.
- It does not merely 'match' other's expressions, as in correspondence, but is nevertheless informed by such meanings.
- Through a body-based hermeneutic process, the understanding becomes aesthetically alive.
- Such 'aliveness' is a pattern of understanding that is connected to both 'otherness' and the 'self'.
- New words or rearranged old words 'come from there' and are offered as potentially applicable and transferable to others for their own hospitality so that they can make temporary 'homes' for such understanding.
- Such understanding has experiential effects and can be used as a lively and intricate experiential reference that can 'check' against all previous expressions including the informants, the researchers and others. This can help one to understand 'more' and 'heartfully' *rather* than the achieving of a correspondent understanding. It has a 'retrospective richness'.
- Understanding is enriched by such 'crossing' and cannot therefore be reduced to a simple summary or one person's formulation. "The crossing of two junctures does not bring the lowest common denominator but rather a great deal that is new to both of the two [understandings] that cross." (Gendlin, 2004b, p. 135). And further: ". . . this can enrich and complicate the earlier findings. But this never makes them wrong or useless." (Gendlin, 2004b, p. 139).
- But more than all of this, this kind of understanding is aesthetically inclusive and carries bodily felt implications.
- Poetic language is helpful within such aesthetically inclusive understanding in that words are 'experiential directions' rather than 'summative descriptors'. Understanding goes beyond the form of the expression.

> Words mean the change they make when they are said . . . when we do not understand a statement, we can only repeat the statement. We repeat its form of words. But when we understand the statement, we can speak from it in many ways.
>
> (Gendlin, 2004b, p. 141)

So phenomenology can re-present words in other ways, and fruitfully draws on a body-based hermeneutics that cares for the aliveness that words can carry forward. From all of the above, it can be seen that Gendlin's notion of 'carrying forward' does not prioritise language in itself nor the bodily sense of 'more than words can say' in itself. Rather, it is interested in the vibrant tension and relationship between words and the bodily felt sense, and the way that both language and the body move together in meaningful ways.

Therefore in pursuing a more aesthetic phenomenology in practice, we arrive at the following principle: the aliveness of language and the empathic use of language to facilitate an experience of homecoming for others.

This emphasis is shared by other qualitative researchers who are moving towards a more aesthetic emphasis and there is an emerging body of literature that considers the value of transforming qualitative research findings in different ways, such as dramatic presentation and evocative writing (Sandelowski, 1998; Spry, 2001; Willis, 2005).

The particular innovation of embodied interpretation, however, develops Gendlin's (1991) philosophy of 'entry into the implicit' and the way in which a more aesthetic phenomenology needs the lived body to facilitate interpretation as a textured practice that is alive with 'more than words can say'. Gendlin goes back to what he considers to be an important concept in Heidegger's work: how feeling is a form of understanding. Gendlin also shows how the body as it lives and feels is a crucial faculty for a form of holistic knowing that is essentially aesthetic. Although this form of knowing can *find* words, it is *larger* than words, because the lifeworld is more than any category of already patterned knowing. In this view, the lifeworld comes in its excess before it is patterned or interpreted.

So Gendlin's contributions focus on the relationship between language and the aliveness or excess of what language was trying to represent or point to. This is a practice rather than a mere 'thinking about', in that such immersion needs the whole body – its senses and feelings. Gendlin calls this the 'felt sense'. A felt sense carried in the lived body faces two ways: it faces the 'more' of the lived world and it faces the possibility of language. The phrase 'entry into the implicit' means that the words that are formulated come from an experiential practice based on attending to the lived body's sense of felt meaning in any moment.

Gendlin was afraid that, in our Cartesian tradition, we would become prematurely abstract in the ways that we categorise and divide up our experience, because this is what words do. Gendlin, like Heidegger, is very respectful of the role of words in understanding – if language is given its proper place. For Gendlin, it is the lived body as it holistically participates in its living, feeling and moving that provides the experiential ground of what words are about. The lived body always knows something about how it finds itself in relation to the more of the lifeworld. It is experiential before it is logical or made into a pattern through reflection and language. Yet, even though it is not articulate in its lively experience, it is in a sense faithful or authentic in that it is in touch with something in an aesthetic way. Merleau-Ponty (1964) spoke of how the lived is greater than the known. The 'lived' in this perspective is then much more encompassing as a faculty of partici-pative knowing than our reflective capacities alone.

Towards an application of these more embodied concerns

Embodied interpretation builds on the previous epistemological framework that draws on both Gadamer and Gendlin. Embodied interpretation has been developed as a way of translating research findings so that health care professionals can be more sensitised to the human dimensions of what it is like to live with different health related conditions and concerns. We thus wish to contribute to methodologies that may help health care professionals to find the 'I' in the 'Thou' of their patients. Within this spirit we aim to offer a methodological innovation that can translate health related research findings in more engaging and emotionally captivating ways.

Embodied interpretation is a body-based hermeneutics in which qualitative meanings are pursued by a back and forth movement between words and their felt complexity in the lived body. This movement between the whole of the felt complexity at any moment (that is 'in the more') and the part that 'comes to language' is a practice that keeps open the creative tension between words and the aliveness of what the words are about.

When, as researchers, we have a digested understanding of what we have heard, perhaps from a number of people, how do we then use this under-standing in our analysis and writing? Giorgi (1997) has written about how it is important to get a sense of the whole of a text or expression so that its details can find their meaningful context. But where is this sense of the whole of an understanding carried by the researcher? Gendlin (1978) would say that it is carried in the body as a background understanding to check against as one writes and analyses. So, as qualitative researchers, our own sense of the 'more' is used to communicate this sense to the readers. We then present com-municatively helpful shapes that are transferable and can deepen under-standing in others. In this process, we have at least two aims:

- To enter the experience and find our own bodily understanding of the whole and of the parts of what has been understood.
- To re-emerge into language so that we can share the insights and com-municate them to others, not only in faithful and rigorous ways but in evocative ways that can awaken the aliveness of the meanings for the reader.

This does not mean that the reader has the same experience as the informants, but that the reader can relate to the understandings in personal and unique ways. To revisit Gadamer (1975/1997), such qualitative understanding is always an intersection of other and self.

The process of embodied interpretation

As in other phenomenological research, we interview a number of people and transcribe what they have said. The practice of embodied interpretation begins after a more traditional scientific phase where the essential narrative structure of the experience is described and presented for readers, similar to the way one would present the findings in Giorgi's (1997) descriptive phenomenological approach. The essential narrative structure is then supplemented by a phase of embodied interpretation. This supplemental practice of embodied interpretation requires us, as researchers, to go back and forth between our embodied sense of the meanings conveyed in the structure and our search for words that can evocatively communicate these meanings. In this way, we are interested in serving public understanding through words that reflect the excess and the aliveness of what our participants have shown us. In a sense, this is not radically different from the way humans interpret and communicate in their everyday lives when they are trying to put emotionally relevant experiences into words. However, Gendlin (1996) has noted a difference between putting things into words with reference to 'bodily alive meanings' and other moments of speaking when we do not connect as much with our bodily felt sense. It is with reference to this body of work that we have reflected on the stages of embodied interpretation.

The process is not linear but a back and forth engagement with the text that is at times muddy and murky, but which works palpably. This back and forth engagement includes the following emphases:

- Being present to others' stories.
- Entry into the alive meanings.
- Dwelling and holding so that meanings can form.
- Finding words that work.

These stages overlap but each is discreet enough to show itself as a necessary emphasis. The stages may be considered meaningful in that they allow the practitioner of embodied interpretation to slow down and 'be with' the communicated phenomena in an embodied way while being open to language. In this process we engage in the practice of focusing (Gendlin, 1981), in which we attend to our own body's felt sense of the meaning of the text. We cannot do justice in this chapter to the complexity of nuanced instructions that have been developed to aid this process, but here describe the broad outline and spirit of the process. For more detailed considerations about such forms of empathising, listening, and bodily engaging with meanings, we refer readers to the large body of work concerning focusing technique (http://www. focusing.org.).

We become bodily open to, and resonant with, the words of our informants as we read the narrative structure. We focus on our own bodily sense of what comes and write down these initial experiences of engaging in such body-based, empathic imagination – it is about paying attention to what the presence of the communicated phenomenon is like when we stand before it in an embodied way. We then go back to the narrative structure, focusing on the details of the text and checking those details against our bodily felt sense: whether they confirm or resonate with the bodily felt sense, or whether the details change the bodily felt sense. If the details change the bodily felt sense, then we write some words or phrases that capture the felt change of this sense. We may go back and forth a number of times until we get a feeling of aesthetic satisfaction that the words are good enough to carry forward the aliveness of the meanings. We then rework the interpretation so that our emerging writing can reflect both the evocative resonance of the text as a whole movement, as well as the breadth and depth of the details. A viable stopping point is arrived at logically, but also aesthetically or bodily respon-sively. This whole movement that goes between the researchers' own bodily felt sense and the text is not just to satisfy the researchers' predilections and traditions of aesthetic preference and understanding. More than this, the aim of the process is to re-enliven the phenomenon for public purposes. Ultimately the real test is therefore its impact on readers and audiences. However, by the researchers first going through a process that enlivens the phenomenon for them, it is perhaps more likely that readers can engage with the results of this more evocative offering in new and emotionally receptive ways. This is consistent with the rationale of any phenomenological explication as an outcome of research which seeks not just to represent details and peoples' words, but to re-present a digested sense of 'wholes' that make the descriptions more relevant to others at an existential level. Churchill (2007, p. 8) refers to this capacity of phenomenological research as '*connectedness*': ". . . the methods employed would be predicated upon a *sensitivity* to meanings requiring some form of direct existential contact between the researcher and the phenomenon."

For an illustration of how we transform an excerpt of a traditional phenomenological analysis (essential narrative structure) into a more evocative re-presentation through the method of 'embodied interpretation', please see Chapter 4. There, we re-present the findings of a study of caring for a life-long partner with Alzheimer's disease in such a way as to emphasise the possibilities of its felt understanding for readers. As such, readers are offered two readings of the findings in Chapter 4: a phenomenological description (Giorgi, 1997; Giorgi & Giorgi, 2003a, 2003b) followed by its transformation into evocative prose. We are arguing that this may facilitate a form of understanding in the reader that appeals to both the head and the heart. This approach is also further illustrated in Chapter 10. There, readers are offered embodied interpretations of findings from three published qualitative research studies in relation to the experience of recovery from a stroke.

Palpable pointing: The value of embodied interpretation

The purpose of this chapter was to primarily introduce the practice of embodied interpretation, and to consider its possible relevance and value. An important question is whether a phase of embodied interpretations adds any value to the way findings are presented. We believe that its added value is that it expands understanding to include the more heart-related dimensions that are central to the empathic imagination. As such, our rationale is to communicate findings in more evocative ways that may support the more participative forms of knowing what a phenomenon may be like, and this requires evocatively impactful language. The value of such empathic under-standing is a kind of knowledge that is not so much about new information (new contributions to propositional knowledge), but about the possibility of enhancing the emotional intelligence of audiences. This may be particularly important in the human sciences, where putting an experience together as an embodied whole may serve as an important intuitive reference to support acting in caring and ethical ways. In finding a way to be faithful to descriptions, and expressing this in more heartfelt ways, the prose of embodied interpretations may help to make an experiential phenomenon more present so that it can live in ways that exceed any summary and find a meaningful relationship with readers' own lives; it is the kind of knowledge that 'touches'. The readers themselves may best judge the extent to which this works for them. Such resonant validity is not about correspondence but about whether the embodied interpretation *carries forward* the general phenomenological structure into the embodied shared horizons, where we can meet in under-standing in plausible and insightful ways. This means that such resonant validity is always 'on the way' and is never complete, because different readers apply the understandings to their own circumstances and concerns. Such a view of understanding is consistent with Gadamer's (1975/1997) notion of validity as application, rather than the notion of validity as an abstract unit of agreement that reflects an unambiguous objective reality.

Conclusion

On one hand, embodied interpretation moves away from traditional descriptive phenomenology towards a more aesthetic phenomenology that appeals to the heart. On the other hand, embodied interpretation also appeals to the head in that it does not go as far as poetry in moving away from the storied details of people's narratives.

Embodied interpretation thus locates itself in the middle of the spectrum: it makes use of the values and power of poetic language to palpably point, but is presented as prose that incorporates a thick description of sequences and concrete details. This is because, not only do we want to be evocative: we also wish to pay attention to a hermeneutic concern that allows sufficient contextual details to show up in the textured prose. Moustakas (1994) expresses similar ideas about how a presentation of phenomenological findings carries elements of both poetic and rational concerns. He has given some clues as to how the presentation of phenomenological findings needs to be more like prose than poetry, in that it should have a structure that gives sufficient detail and context.

Finally, we would like to suggest that by reading both the essential narrative structure of the phenomenological analysis *and* the more evocative sense of the embodied interpretations, carers, professionals, family and support groups could be better equipped to understand and respond to 'what people go through' in their poignant journeys in relation to well-being and suffering. In this way such re-presentations of qualitative research findings could meaningfully facilitate the kinds of embodied relational understandings that serve the empathic imagination and the heartfelt capacity to care.

12 Embodying nursing open-heartedness

An illustration of a core capacity for caring

At the end of the day, the practice of caring is a form of 'living' and not just a matter of 'knowing'. Yet caring as a living practice does include certain kinds of knowing and understanding as indicated previously. This is why in the last three chapters we have concentrated on the kinds of epistemologies that are conducive to caring, and in this context, we emphasised the notions of embodied relational understanding, the empathic imagination, and the kinds of research-based knowledge that can speak to the heart of caring and the heart of practice.

In this chapter we would like to indicate how the practice of caring is not just a matter of knowing, nor a matter of mere instrumental application. Rather, it is a matter of the 'living' of the 'open heart'. We wish to show how this *capacity* to keep the heart open, to embody this in one's practice, is sometimes a matter of knowing, is sometimes a matter of 'not knowing', but is essentially expressed as an integrated and holistic capacity for care.

We consider these issues in relation to the practice of nursing because we believe nursing practice offers a good example of the kinds of complex, marginal and holistic situations where the need for 'open-heartedness' is often enacted. We aim to articulate and illustrate this phenomenon that we have called 'nursing open-heartedness' as a foundational resource for acting in caring ways. As such we wish to articulate what is distinctive about nursing 'open-heartedness,' not only philosophically but also in a style that can evoke the lived sense of its meaning. Our contention is that the phenomenon we wish to articulate as 'nursing open-heartedness' is central to the phenomenon of caring. We wish to show that nursing open-heartedness is more complex than just an empathic encounter, that it makes use of the procedural but is not determined by it, and that it faces vulnerabilities of being human without excessive minimisation on the one hand, or excessive romanticising on the other.

A number of nursing theorists have considered how the phenomenon of caring is central to the philosophy of nursing and have offered theoretical frameworks for nursing care (Chaska, 1990; Chinn & Kramer, 1999; Newman, 1994, 1999; Parse, 1981; Rogers, 1980; Watson, 1996, 2011). Central to these theories is a holistic concern to reflect ontologies and epistemologies that can do justice to the practice of nursing in a non-reductionist way (Drew & Dahlberg, 1995). Dahlberg and Drew (1997) offer a lifeworld perspective based on the phenomenological tradition to describe five dimensions that are important for conceptualising holistic nursing and one of these is 'open-mindedness and open-heartedness'. Although their consideration of open-heartedness focuses most on its implication for a holistic research approach, the emphasis on availability to others and "the capacity to be surprised and sensitive to the unpredictable and unexpected" (p. 306) are important dimensions for holistic care as well. Birx (2003) has been influential for us in considering the relationship between holistic nursing and open-heartedness, drawing on her significant experiences and studies in the Zen tradition. Although acknowledging the contributions of all these theorists and practitioners, our focus in this chapter is not to enter into a critical analysis of this body of work, but to offer a novel and distinctive way of understanding the phenomenon of 'nursing open-heartedness'.

We do so by going back to some seminal continental philosophers for inspiration, and attempt to illustrate the insights derived through a number of imaginative vignettes from practice. We focus on the phenomenon of 'nursing open-heartedness' for three reasons. First, in our philosophical enquiries we became interested in the *source* of caring as a focus rather than on caring per se. Second, guided by the continental philosophical tradition, we became interested in what it is in our capacities as human beings that enables care. In the work of Levinas, although he did not use the term, we found a view of 'open-heartedness' in general that potentially comes with the territory of being human. Third, we then became interested in whether there was anything distinctive about nursing open-heartedness as a particular variation or nuance of open-heartedness in general. This led to further elaboration drawing on other relevant continental philosophers. But there is also a more pragmatic reason why we wish to focus on 'nursing open-heartedness': we believe, with others, that nursing care is in danger of being commodified within an increasingly instrumental 'audit culture' (Cooley, 2004; Nortvedt, 1996, 2001; Pask, 2005; Young, 2000, cited in Young, 2002). Therefore such nursing open-heartedness may be important as the humanising face of procedural, instrumental or technical knowledge. Within this understanding, nursing open-heartedness is the meaningful human context within which technical knowledge can be integrated and applied. Our hope is to share and communicate this phenomenon in both a philosophically interesting, as well as an evocative way that allows a 'felt' sense of its significance and potential application in practice. Such a style of theory building attempts to be logical but, in addition, moves towards a more contemplative and experiential direction. As such we arrive at a view of 'nursing open-heartedness' that is constituted by three essential dimensions.

We proceed by presenting three vignettes of nursing situations that raise particular questions regarding the challenges for nurses of responding in humanly caring ways. These concrete circumstances provide a context within which to discuss the complexity of nursing open-heartedness and we show how it shares important dimensions with open-heartedness in general.

In this task we draw upon and are centrally informed by important insights from the philosophical works of Emmanuel Levinas, Maurice Merleau-Ponty, and Martin Heidegger. We integrate some of their philosophical insights to show how these can be used to throw light on the essence of open-heartedness in nursing. From this, the following three dimensions of nursing open-heartedness are described:

- The infinity of otherness: keeping open the other's difference.
- Embodiment: our shared vulnerable heritage.
- Practical responsiveness: embracing the value of the objectified gaze and technology.

However, despite separating out these three dimensions for clarity, we would like to emphasise how these dimensions essentially interrelate to create the complex space within which the open-hearted nurse functions. This complex space embodies both the simple 'givenness' of the open heart or 'song of innocence' that comes with the vicissitudes of being human, and an openness to the complex skills and training or 'song of experience' that comes with personal and professional development (Blake, 1794/2008). Building on this, open-heartedness is therefore something that needs to be opened up and sustained rather than built up or instilled from scratch as if it were not already a part of being human.

We move on to examine the implications of our description of nursing open-heartedness for personal development in practice. Gendlin's (1991, 1997a, 1997b) 'Philosophy of Entry into the Implicit' is used as a way of understanding how nursing open-heartedness can be embodied within our everyday experiences. The chapter concludes by providing some particular directions for highlighting nursing open-heartedness as an important embodied resource for everyday practice.

The challenges of nursing open-heartedness revealed in three clinical encounters

The following vignettes give examples of practice situations that nurses might experience during everyday practice. We would like to emphasise that in choosing these vignettes and the way the nurse responds in each case we are not recommending the solution the nurse reaches as the best or only prescription for action, as if this is how nursing open-heartedness 'should be' or 'look like'. Rather in these vignettes we want to consider the process, rather than the particular outcome. As such, the nurses in their own unique way are negotiating an awareness of the dimension that we wish to illustrate. So it is not the specificity of the particular action that we wish to most illustrate but the nature of the dimension as it appears, and is engaged with by the nurse in some way.

Vignette 1: Death scene

The scenario is a death bed. It is not a peaceful scene. The room is brightly lit and it is a hot day outside in the garden. The young woman of 22 is fighting for air; she is angry and her young but broken body, savaged by chemotherapy, is fighting to live as it is dying. Each breath brings a rasp, a low, throated gasp which signals her determination to fight . . . to hold on to her rapid breathing. The nurse standing at the bedside is the same age; her task is to be present. The nurse can feel the young woman's anger, her bitter fight; she identifies with it, but she also senses that it is not her anger because she is not the other. There is a boundary between her own body and the dying body before her, but the nurse is still intensely frightened. She can imagine her own frailty, she senses a quickening in the pit of her stomach; she feels a deep gut-wrenching futility, the overpowering uncertainty of her own body, her life, that 'this could be me'. At the same time she remains deeply frightened for the young woman and she stays close to her.

So what keeps open an interaction that can bear the helplessness of this plight? What kind of open-heartedness can bear the possibility of the other not having a 'good death'? This vignette confronts us with the challenge of opening to an extreme example of the *infinity of otherness* (Levinas 1974/1981), a term that we will explore later as being one of the three core dimensions of the essences of nursing open-heartedness. This is the first challenge that we wish to explore in articulating the essence of nursing open-heartedness.

Vignette 2: Humiliation scene

The scenario is faecal incontinence. A man of 45 is laid on his back in a hospital bed on an open ward with seven other patients. It is the middle of the day and meals are about to be served. He is lying in his faeces and he is in pain. He cannot move and is aware of the stench of his faeces and the presence of other patients. He has been like this for five minutes but he knows the nurse is on his way – he has gone to get a bowl, cloths and water. He feels a degree of self-disgust, even self-loathing; an overpowering anxiety, a deep worry that everyone around is also extremely averse to this situation and is bearing this smell resentfully. He wants to be invisible, not noticed.

So what keeps open an interaction that carries a humanising quality that is appropriate to this poignancy? What kind of open-heartedness can bear the possibility of the other's extreme vulnerability and shame? This vignette confronts us with the challenge of opening to an extreme example of our shared heritage, our vulnerable body. This is the second challenge that we wish to explore in articulating the essence of nursing open-heartedness and we will later explore embodiment (Merleau-Ponty 1964/1968) as being a further core dimension of the essence of nursing open-heartedness.

Vignette 3: Ambivalence scene

The man is 50 years old. His arms are maimed with a multitude of deep scars arranged almost neatly, as if following the creases in the pattern of a jumper sleeve. He is bleeding badly from a new wound and he has been drinking. The cut is deep and precise. The man tells the nurse that he has been fighting against the urge to cut for about a week, since he was released from prison. He does not like coming into contact with health services and has only attended because the cut is deep. He carries with him a troubled history of punitive care at the hands of some professionals in the past. At other times, some well-meaning and respectful professionals have tried to leave him alone and he then ended up in hospital after another episode of self-cutting.

So what keeps open an interaction that can be simply responsive at different levels, from deeply existential to exceedingly practical and interventionist? What kind of open-heartedness is free from ideological or personal agendas and carries an ability that moves with the occasion? This vignette confronts us with the challenge of opening to an extreme example where the other's survival is dependent on technical intervention, and which requires the value of an objectified gaze. How is this objectified gaze included in open-heartedness? This is the third challenge that we wish to explore in articulating the essence of nursing open-heartedness and we will later explore the concept of 'readiness to hand' (Heidegger 1927/1962) as an additional core dimension of the essence of nursing open-heartedness.

We now offer responses to each of the three challenges as a way of moving towards an articulation of what is distinctive about the essence of nursing open-heartedness.

The challenges of nursing open-heartedness

The infinity of otherness: Keeping open the other's difference

One of Levinas's (1969/1987) central insights is that subjectivity arises from a traumatic exposure to alterity (the other). Therefore, the meeting between nurse and patient is not simply an empathic encounter based on commonality or sameness. The other person can never be reduced to what one knows, defined by one's familiar ideas. The infinity or alterity of otherness is much more ambiguous than any judgement or conclusion that we may need to latch on to for the sake of security or belonging. An acknowledgement of such alterity beyond oneself is a demand to grant freedom to what is other than oneself. This is an important dimension of nursing open-heartedness.

When faced in open-heartedness, Vignette 1 announces the extreme alone-ness of another's imminent death with its angry or shocking struggle to 'not go gently into the dying of the light'. The nurse, who is the same age, may already be faced with a sense of the irrevocable transition from the remembered aliveness of her patient to a lifeless corpse, seen there on the bed. Such otherness may be so threateningly alien that the nurse withdraws from any relationship with such otherness. It would be easiest here for the nurse to take refuge in a voyeuristic stance of the fascination of 'not me in there . . . I am part of the well-world'. This voyeuristic stance flees from a relationship with otherness to a relation with the more comfortable 'we-world' of excluding otherness. Another possible response by the nurse may be to 'busy about' in a professional manner distracting oneself while the other is dying, leaving the dying one alone in the gravity of her situation.

In open-heartedness, the nurse can never fully know the gravity of the dying and the death of another, but she can allow herself this 'not knowing' and be addressed by whatever the concreteness of this moment seems to humanly require. This is an important part of the story of nursing open-heartedness, but we also need to say something about our primordial human connected-ness. And here we come to Merleau-Ponty and embodiment.

Embodiment: Our shared vulnerable heritage

Nursing open-heartedness is particularly exercised when confronted with bodily suffering, the body's dominance as an object, its levelling power. This is the fundamental source of our shared heritage: the fleshly ground that binds us and out of which we come. Such embodied intertwining opens us to a shared vulnerability and possible reversibility with others. One of Merleau-Ponty's (1945/1962) central insights is that human beings are both body object and body subjects. Merleau-Ponty differentiated these two perspectives of the body in order to indicate how we can regard our body at different times: on the one hand as if it was an objective 'thing' independent of ourselves and, at other times, as a body subject whose meanings are lived and felt from within.

In Vignette 2 the nurse is called to respond with more than a perfunctory, safe distant 'clean up' as if cleaning an inanimate object. The skilled and open-hearted nurse will approach the bed space and the patient in a way that does not exhibit a wall of denial. Nor will the nurse express a distant, objective task-orientation, a cold robotic approach to the intervention that would add to the shame of the patient. The nurse does not just regard the patient as a body object by infantilising him as if he were a baby. Nor does he objectify him by depersonalising him and treating him as if no-one is there, just a collection of instrumental body parts. Instead, he may be open to a sense of both his own and the patient's vulnerability.

At the same time, such acknowledgement is not simply a felt awareness of our shared subjective bodies. An awareness of our vulnerable heritage also encompasses an acknowledgement of our shared body objects. This ambiguous embodied heritage regarding the possible reversibility between body subject and body object makes possible an openness to act in a way that mediates the self-disgust and public humiliation experienced with the more factual vicissitudes of body parts beyond control. Such open-heartedness to the complexity of embodiment thus acknowledges both body as carnal matter and body as soulful window to the depth of a life. This is a powerful and respectful 'intimate distance' in the context of a sensitively delivered task to change the linen and wash the patient's body. The bodily care will be gentle but not overly drawn out. It will aim to bring physical comfort speedily. Perhaps there may be 'just the right amount' of conversation mixed with the sound of water: "This won't take long . . . I know it is not OK . . . as you get stronger this won't happen, it is just your body saying I am really tired and sick right now". So this vignette announces a certain poignancy of our most basic primal and private physical contingencies.

An open-heartedness to the nature of embodiment in both self and other may therefore be particularly important in nursing. The nurse sees our bodily predicaments as a shared heritage and as such can meet the person there. This is an important part of the story of nursing open-heartedness, but we need to say something even more strongly about the practicality of nursing open-heartedness, which we illustrate with reference to our third vignette. We turn now to Heidegger (1927/1962) and his practical notion of openness – what he calls 'readiness to hand'.

Practical responsiveness: Embracing the value of the objectified gaze and technology

One of Heidegger's (1927/1962) central philosophical contributions concerns how 'knowing how to be' in different situations does not primarily come from abstract or theoretical reflection, but essentially emerges out of a very practical engagement with people, things and situations as they happen. He has called this dimension 'Zuhandensein' or 'readiness to hand'. The fertile possibilities for action are very specific in that the unique circumstances of any moment are always more complex than any generalisation, categorisation or 'knowing in advance'. With this emphasis in mind, open-heartedness is very practical in that it responds from within the relational complexity of the situation rather than from a preconceived self-position. In such open-heartedness, one is then somewhat free from ideological or personal agendas to be more freely responsive to the occasion. This may include forms of preconceived diagnoses or routine ways of acting – such as from policies and guidelines – for certain categories of patients or needs.

One may think that open-minded practical responsiveness is naïve in that it is so open to novel nuances in a situation. However, it is also open to all the historical and technical resources that are available from one's specialised training and life experience. So this kind of practical responsiveness is free to draw on the value of the objectified gaze and any technological resources if that is what is called for. This dimension of practical responsive open-heartedness, however, appropriately uses the value of the objectified gaze where necessary rather than being defined by it. Without this open-heartedness, the objectified gaze and technology could easily become ways of depersonalising others. Practically responsive open-heartedness thus embraces the value of the 'procedural' but is not determined by it.

In relation to this, Vignette 3 highlights the patient's deeply anguished existence but also the more immediate priority of 'fixing up' his arm. The nurse's technical expertise to suture the wound is drawn upon in a quick and efficient manner. Here, a nurse may find it easier to indulge in a judgemental attitude that takes the moral high ground of deeming the patient to be not quite deserving of care. Or the nurse may become overly involved in the anguish of the other, overstepping the tacit request by the patient to simply be met for now at an instrumental level.

So what 'keeps open' an interaction that understands that open-heartedness is not necessarily 'saintly' but can be simply responsive at different levels, from deeply existential to exceedingly practical? Here the nurse has the confidence to trust the spontaneity of what comes next. She is able to embody a sufficient degree of not knowing in advance. Such an encounter means entering ambiguity and unpredictability but then to also be available to all the specialised and technical resources to hand. In the practical responsiveness of open-heartedness, a technical rational perspective has a value and purpose when it serves the very concrete need, whether this is for care or cure.

This is an important part of the story of nursing open-heartedness but we also need to say something about how the emphases of 'otherness', 'embodiment' and 'practicality' are already integrated and come together within the essence of nursing open-heartedness.

The essence of nursing open-heartedness: Being there for otherness, embodiment and practical responsiveness

Nursing open-heartedness is particularly exercised in profiles of bodily dominance, finitude and marginality. These are the nursing 'places' where the three dimensions of otherness, embodiment and practicality all cohere. Here is an embodied person who calls us in both our sameness and difference, in a practical concrete moment that is always more complex than we can name. Nursing open-heartedness, in embracing the three dimensions in its essence, is not a static state but a fluid phenomenon in which the three dimensions are mutually present but with different emphases and relationships at different times. In this ambiguous space, the three dimensions are intertwined but offer distinctive nuances.

Such openness holds an ambiguity that straddles bodily matter and person: although a person's physical presence may be wretched, this does not obscure the sense of the person who is there. Such openness does not exist in an esoteric, ideological realm. It is much more sober and concrete, and there is a call to the human heart. It is an openness to situations of disjunction, powerlessness and weakness; of facing these vulnerabilities without minimising them on one hand or romanticising them on the other. Such openness is functionally intelligent and straddles both instrumental expertise and non-purposive 'meeting' or 'presence'. It is a form of giving that 'gets the fit right'. It can respect the appropriateness of the instrumental but remains open to both the shining vital person as well as to the body-object that is skin, muscle and bone. So this openness is free from agenda and spontaneously gives what is needed, from the very practical to the most existential. It can travel the range with a particular kind of fluidity. In all these ways, nursing open-heartedness is a 'primordial act of hospitality' (Jager, 2001). But we would like to say something more about the complexity of this primordial act of hospitality, its source and its challenge.

Songs of innocence and experience

The givenness of open-heartedness and its challenge to survive in complex and marginal situations

The givenness and source of open-heartedness is deeply embedded in our intrinsic awareness of, and call to, the other's vulnerability. Levinas (1969/1987) sees this as a very pre-reflective and spontaneous gesture that is given to human beings before they learn to cover this over with guardedness, self-defence or the need to attack. Such primordial open-heartedness in Levinas's sense does not need to be cultivated from scratch but rather needs to be uncovered. If this source of open-heartedness is primordially given with relationality, and is therefore in a certain sense innocent, how can such open-heartedness be kept open in such a way as to meet the complexities of nursing practice? How do such songs of innocence survive the songs of experience?

So far we have articulated nursing open-heartedness as a complex sensitivity that is open to the infinity of otherness, the vulnerability of our shared embodied heritage and the practical responsiveness that flexibly moves, depending on what is needed, from the highly specialised and technical to the most spontaneous and uniquely personal. This complex sensitivity requires a certain fluidity and 'play' between all these dimensions (responsiveness, including specialised knowing and technology, otherness, and embodiment). Its complexity thus needs the benefits of both 'songs of innocence' and 'songs of experience'; it is not merely a simple openness to the innocence of a naïve heart. Nursing open-heartedness therefore requires both integration of nursing life experience as well as a fluidity of what is uncovered in our intrinsic awareness of human vulnerability. In the context of everyday practice, such an integrative sense of nursing open-heartedness is fragile and easily lost. One could either become hardened by experience or lost and overwhelmed by the innocence of the open heart. The challenge is then one of how to hold on to this kind of understanding that comes from an integrated awareness of the infinity of otherness, the vulnerability of our shared embodied heritage and the practical responsiveness that flexibly moves. Such holding on to this kind of understanding is much more important than anything else one can *do*. Indeed, rushing to do something may reduce the clarity of the under-standing or even obscure it altogether. Rather, directions for action arise more credibly by 'coming from' the stance of integrated understanding.

The philosopher and psychologist Eugene Gendlin, in his philosophy of 'Entry into the Implicit', elaborates on the kind of understanding that is embodied and which can form an authentic but tacit guide for action. Other authors who have written about embodied understanding in slightly different ways are Polanyi's (1996) view of tacit understanding, Benner' s (1984) contributions to the nature of integrated expert practice, Logstrup's (1995, 1997) embodied sensing, and Todres's (2007) approach to 'embodied enquiry'. Within this spirit, we draw on Gendlin's consideration of the impor-tance of a kind of understanding that brings together 'head', 'hand' and 'heart' (understanding, application and feeling), which is particularly relevant to the notion of practical wisdom (*phronesis*). To aid the development of 'lived understandings' that are not just theoretical but that are embodied and can inform practice, Gendlin has developed practical guidance for achieving such integrated lived understandings, through the approach he calls 'focusing' (Gendlin, 1981): "Focusing is a process of finding 'felt senses', being friendly to them, symbolizing them, and allowing them to shift" (Friedman, 2000, p. 69). A felt sense is a bodily way of knowing something before it becomes explicit and named; for example, like the whole sense of how things are between myself and my partner or co-worker. The felt sense is the way we bodily experience meanings that are implicit in our relationship to situations, people and things. It is a way in which our more abstract ways of knowing are implicitly connected to more personal and unique experiences that make them meaningful. In this way we are able to hold meanings in our body as a holistic felt sense of these meanings that have relevance for our lives (see Gendlin, 1981, and http://www.focusing.org). Consistent with this view, the most essential thing we can do as a direction for practice is the sensing and holding of an embodied understanding of nursing open-heartedness. So, the capacity to sustain the complexity of nursing open-heartedness is about accessing, remembering or being 'grabbed by' lived experiences that are felt touchstones for the three dimensions of nursing open-heartedness. The importance of these experiential touchstones is the direction they give to everyday nursing activity. Many actions can flow from this but, in the spirit of this enquiry, we would not like to specify these possible actions because this would obscure the essential gesture or comportment of embodied understanding. Embodied understanding involves a living access to important feelings and insights that are carried and affirmed and are more than just principles, or abstract thoughts.

Nursing open-heartedness: Towards personal development for practice

There is much that has been written and which could still be written about the power of institutional, political and structural contexts that act to diminish or obscure the practice of nursing open-heartedness (for example Barnett, 2005; Benner, 2000; Foucault, 1973; Frank, 2004; Goffman, 1968; Komesaroff, 2001; Melia, 1987). We acknowledge that all of these conditions need attention. In this particular chapter, however, we are concentrating on articulating the existential character of nursing open-heartedness as a touchstone from where these institutional, political and structural contexts could be negotiated. We thus leave this larger task of considering these broader contexts that may challenge or support open-heartedness for a future project. For now we would like to conclude by offering a way of tapping into an embodied sense of experience that can become a resource for practice in ongoing ways. We do this by means of a fourth vignette that portrays an indication of such an embodied resource.

Vignette 4

Rueben is nurse who is providing home-based care for Lilly, an older frail person who is bedridden, needs artificial feeding and has a catheter. Rueben has been visiting Lilly every day for the past four weeks. Today, Lilly has a very severe chest infection, cannot tolerate any feeding and is dehydrated. Rueben does not know this yet. He walks into Lilly's bedroom; she looks over at him, clearly distressed in some way but unable to talk. There is an appeal in her eyes that communicates an immediate mix of human predicaments: distress at the struggle to draw the next breath, a restless discomfort that can't find escape, a direct look at Rueben which says: 'I can't go on, can you help me?'

Time slows down for Rueben. He sees all of this without yet categorising or knowing what is happening specifically to her in a technical way at this stage. From somewhere deep within him there is a bodily recognition of the marginality of her desperate struggle and appeal. It is in excess of any words. Yet he knows something about that, whether it is on an existential level, as part of the history of being human (for instance as a struggling baby exposed to the dawning life-threatening necessity to breathe), or whether on a more personal level relevant to his more unique history (such as, a time when he could not swim as a five-year-old and his parents were out of sight). It is not the specific details of these experiences that are important here but how they announce a sense of being in a bodily marginal and vulnerable space. He does not necessarily consciously recall these existential and personal incidents of bodily vulnerability. Rather he has a felt sense as a fellow human being who knows something about the nature of bodily desperation and marginality. At this stage, however, Rueben is simply and innocently there as a human being who knows the meaning of desperate marginal vulnerability, not just as a bystander but as a participant in a shared human existence.

We leave the vignette at this stage to consider how Rueben's implicit knowing in his body can become a resource for remembering and highlighting nursing open-heartedness. Rueben knows in an embodied way something about the 'shared vulnerability' dimension of open-heartedness. In a sense it was uncovered for him and 'grabbed' him. We could have developed similar vignettes about other nurses' experiences that emphasise the 'otherness' dimension or the 'responsive' dimension of nursing open-heartedness. However, this vignette may be sufficient to reflect upon the question of how such everyday experiences, in very unique ways, may be used as a resource. In this view, embodied experiences function as a way of remembering and acting from an implicit felt experience of open-heartedness in more conscious ways. Such an implicit felt experience that can act as a resource is carried as a 'felt sense' in Gendlin's philosophy. This 'felt sense' is a guide for action that is different and more than a set of thought principles. It is more immediate and holistic in that it includes implicit existential and personal information that draws on what one has lived through. This way of knowing gives it a credibility that is central to linking the personal with the professional. The 'felt sense' as a resource thus serves to make the essences of nursing open-heartedness live in an embodied way. Facilitating the awareness of such embodied understanding may be particularly important if we wish concepts like 'nursing open-heartedness' not to be too abstract, 'academic' or excessively idealistic. Rather such embodied understanding is built on experiences that in a sense are very close to oneself and recognised in their palpable way. Concepts that come from such 'palpability' are thus deemed to offer an important ongoing resource for practice.

Final thoughts

Nursing open-heartedness is an understanding and practice that is developmental and never-ending. However, it is not just based on some abstract ideal of a nurse trying to aspire to using primarily conceptual resources. Rather, human existence is overflowing with embodied experiences that can provide the possibility of an intimate knowing of the kinds of dimensions of nursing open-heartedness that we have articulated in this chapter. To harness such experiences for further development, we may need to find ways of slowing down in such moments, to recognise the value of such experiences, to honour such experiences as resources, and to learn to trust such recognitions as the means to further open, guard and promote the kind of nursing open-heartedness that humanises care.

In articulating the three dimensions of nursing open-heartedness, we hope to have provided a view that practitioners can learn to hold and use as a pointer and a strong experiential basis for personal and professional development as they negotiate the many institutional, political and structural challenges to human-centred practices of care. In considering how nursing open-heartedness is grounded in the existential dimensions of being human, and how these dimensions can be accessed by means of embodied understanding, we offer one view on how nursing open-heartedness may be understood and lived from.

13 Conclusion

Caring for well-being

In this book we have tried to show how lifeworld-oriented philosophy and research, grounded in the phenomenological tradition, can offer valuable ways to approach the phenomena of health-related caring and well-being.

In this respect we have built on other existentially oriented approaches that focus on health, illness, well-being, suffering and caring, such as found in the writings of Boss (1979), Svenaeus (2000), Toombs (1993), Dahlberg (2008), Carel (2008), Benner (1994), Morse (2012), Morse and Johnson (1991), Martinsen (2006), Parse (1984) and others. Our approach shares with them a focus on the seamless and holistic breadth and depth of the lifeworld as a context for understanding human experience, including the more specific variations of human experience within this (illness, well-being, suffering, caring). And particularly in common with Medard Boss (1979), we have found it valuable in relation to health-related caring practices to draw on specific dimensions of the lifeworld (spatiality, temporality, intersubjectivity, embodiment and mood) as providing existential levels of description that are more comprehensive than the narrower biomedical descriptions of what people go through. This has allowed us to offer a 'vocabulary' and a conceptual framework that we believe are sorely needed if care is going to *be* care, and well-being is going to *be* well-being.

But further to Boss we believe that we offer a number of philosophical and research projects relevant to health care that are particularly important at this time. The central theme of these projects can be articulated in the notion 'caring for well-being'. This theme 'caring for well-being' has guided us in the attempt to put some flesh on a number of distinctive but overlapping projects:

- The humanisation of care.
- An articulation of the kinds of well-being that can provide specific and delineated *directions* for care (a focus on well-being resources as a complement to a focus on symptoms and disease processes).
- An articulation of the kinds of suffering that can lead to specific and delineated empathic understandings of the existential depths of 'what people go through' in suffering and illness.

- Epistemological practices that are embodied and not just theoretical or abstract. These places where 'knowing' meets 'being' casts the net wide in disciplinary terms (the arts, the humanities and human sciences) and can serve to intensify the *capacity* for lifeworld-oriented care.

Each of the above projects provides something distinctive to the thematic unifying narrative: caring for well-being. The humanisation of care project addresses the meaning of care and its value. The humanising conceptual framework may further provide some practical strategies with these values in mind. The inclusion of a theory of well-being and suffering, with its delineation of different kinds and levels, provides the *focus* for care. Whereas well-being provides a positive direction (the 'towards' of care), an understanding of suffering can focus carers on the deepest and widest vulnerabilities that call for care. Such understanding of suffering thus serves to widen and intensify the capacity for care. Embodied epistemologies that unify thinking and feeling, knowing and being, also deepen and intensify the capacity for humanly sensitive care in that it is able to stay close and faithful to the qualities of vulnerabilities and freedoms that are the well-springs of care.

Running through all of this is the central existential stance that begins and ends in the non-negotiable fundamentals of living as human beings. And this concern continues to grab us as the challenge to think of health, illness, well-being and suffering not as nouns, but as verbs, never separate from the encompassing lifeworld-flows within which these movements have their meaning.

Our sense of the *whole* of the *movement* of 'caring for well-being' can perhaps underpin a range of possible directions for practice and policy. We would not like to constrain these possibilities, and hesitate to prescribe some of our own particular interests in this regard. Rather, we would like to end by pointing to the central spirit of embodied caring that we believe threads through all the themes we have discussed: the generous hospitality of a meeting place that can authentically call itself human.

References

Abdul-Quader, A.S. (1992). Injecting drug users and female sexual partners of drug users outreach on the Lower East Side of New York city. *British Journal of Addiction*, 81, 681–688.

Abram, D. (1996). *The Spell of the Sensuous: Perception and Language in a More-than-human World*. New York, NY: Vintage Books.

Aggarwal, N., Vass, A.A., Minardi, H.A., Ward, R., Garfield, C. & Cybyk, B. (2003). People with dementia and their relatives: Personal experiences of Alzheimer's and the provision of care. *Journal of Psychiatric and Mental Health Nursing*, 10 (2), 187–197.

AACN [American Association of Colleges in Nursing]. (1999). *Hallmarks of Scholarly Nursing Practice*. Washington, DC: Author.

Arendt, H. (1963). *Eichmann in Jerusalem: A Report on the Banality of Evil*. London, UK: Faber & Faber.

Aristotle. (1983). *Nichomachean Ethics* (T. Irwin, Trans.). Indianapolis, IN: Hackett Publishing Company.

Arman, M., Rannheim, A., Rehnsfeldt, A. & Wode, K. (2008). Anthroposophic healthcare: Different and homelike. *Scandinavian Journal of Caring Science* 22, 357–366.

Ashworth, A. & Ashworth, P. (2003). The lifeworld as phenomenon and as research heuristic, exemplified by a study of the lifeworld of a person suffering Alzheimer's disease. *Journal of Phenomenological Psychology*, 34 (2), 179–205.

Ashworth, P.D. (2003). An approach to phenomenological psychology: The contingencies of the lifeworld. *Journal of Phenomenological Psychology*, 34, 145–156.

Bachelard, G. (1964/2004). *The Poetics of Space* (M. Jolas, Trans.). Boston, MA: Beacon Press.

Barnett, C. (2005). Ways of relating: Hospitality and the acknowledgement of otherness. *Progress in Human Geography*, 29 (1), 5–21.

Basho. (1692–94/2008). *The Complete Haiku* (translated with an introduction biography and notes by Jane Reichhold). London, UK: Kodhansha International.

Bates, M.J. (1989). The design of browsing and berrypicking techniques for the online search interface. *Online Review*, 13 (5), 407–425.

Beck, B., Halling, S., McNabb, M., Miller, D., Rowe, J.O. & Schulz, J. (2003). Facing up to hopelessness: A dialogical phenomenological study. *Journal of Religion and Health*, 42 (4), 339–354.

Beck, C.T. (2001). Caring within nursing education: A metasynthesis. *Journal of Nursing Education,* 40 (3), 101–109.

Benner, P. (1984). *From Novice to Expert.* Reading, MA: Addison-Wesley.

Benner, P. (1994). *Interpretive Phenomenology: Embodiment, Caring and Ethics in Health and Illness.* London, UK: Sage.

Benner, P. (2000). The roles of embodiment, emotion and lifeworld for rationality and agency in nursing practice. *Nursing Philosophy,* 1, 5–19.

Benner, P., & Chesla, C. (1998). *Expertise in Nursing Practice: Caring, Clinical Judgement and Ethics.* New York, NY: Springer.

Benner, P., Hopper-Kyriakidis, P. & Stannard, D. (2010). *Clinical Wisdom and Interventions in Acute and Critical Care: A Thinking-in-Action Approach* (2nd ed.). New York, NY: Springer.

Biley, F.C. & Champney-Smith, A. (2003). "Attempting to say something without saying it . . .": Writing haiku in health care education. *Medical Humanities,* 29, 39–42.

Birx, E. (2003). *Healing Zen: Buddhist Wisdom on Compassion, Caring and Caregiving: For Yourself and Others.* London, UK: Penguin.

Birx, E. (1994). The Poetry of Nursing. *Journal of Holistic Nursing,* 8 (6), 293–303.

Blake, W. (1794/2008). *Songs of Innocence and Songs of Experience.* New York, NY: Dover Publications.

Boss, M. (1963). *Psychoanalysis and Daseinsanalysis.* New York, NY: Basic Books.

Boss, M. (1979). *Existential Foundations of Medicine and Psychology* (S. Conway & A. Cleaves, Trans.). New York, NY: Jason Aronson.

Boyer, E.L. (1990). *Scholarship Reconsidered: Priorities of the Professoriate.* Princeton, NJ: Carnegie Endowment for the Advancement of Teaching.

Bremer, A., Dahlberg, K. & Sandman, L. (2009). To survive out-of hospital cardiac arrest: A search for meaning and coherence. *Qualitative Health Research,* 19, 323–338.

Bretall, R. (Ed.). (1973). *A Kierkegaard Anthology.* Princeton, NJ: Princeton University Press.

Brown, H.I. (1988). *Rationality.* New York, NY: Routledge.

Buber, M. (1970). *I and Thou* (W. Kaufmann, Trans.). Edinburgh, UK: T. & T. Clark.

Buckingham, C.D. & Adams, A. (2000a). Classifying clinical decision making: A unifying approach. *Journal of Advanced Nursing,* 32 (4), 981–989.

Buckingham, C.D. & Adams, A. (2000b). Classifying clinical decision making: Interpreting nursing intuition, heuristic and medical diagnosis. *Journal of Advanced Nursing,* 32 (4), 990–998.

Carel, H. (2008). *Illness: The Cry of the Flesh.* Stocksfield, UK: Acumen.

Carlsson, G., Dahlberg, K., Dahlberg, H. & Ekebergh, M. (2006). Patients longing for authentic personal care: A phenomenological study of violent encounters in psychiatric settings. *Issues in Mental Health Nursing,* 27 (3), 287–305.

Carlsson, G., Dahlberg, K., Lützen, K. & Nyström, M. (2004). Violent encounters in psychiatric care: A phenomenological study of embodied caring knowledge. *Issues in Mental Health Nursing,* 25 (2), 191–217.

Carper, B.A. (1978). Fundamental patterns of knowing in nursing. *Advances in Nursing Science,* 1 (6), 13–23.

Cash, M.A. (2009). *Liberating Qualitative Research Findings Form the Dusty Shelf of Academia: Developing a Translational Methodology Illustrated by a Case Study of the Experience of Living with Dementia.* Unpublished PhD thesis, Bournemouth University, UK.

Chan, Z.C.Y. (2003a). A poem: Anorexia. *Qualitative Inquiry,* 9 (6), 956–957.

Chan, Z.C.Y. (2003b). Poetry writing: A therapeutic means for the social work doctoral student in the process of study. *Journal of Poetry Therapy,* 16 (1), 5–17.

Chan, Z.C.Y. (2010). Reading plays to learn qualitative data analysis: An example of *Death of a Salesman. Journal of Advanced Nursing,* 66 (2), 475–476.

Charmaz, K. (2006). Measuring pursuits, marking self: Meaning construction in chronic illness. *International Journal of Qualitative Studies on Health and Well-being,* 1, 27–37.

Charon, R. (2006). The self-telling body. *Narrative Inquiry,* 16 (1), 191–200.

Chaska, N.L. (1990). *The Nursing Profession: Turning Points.* St Louis, MO: CV Mosby Company.

Chinn, P.L. (Ed.). (1991). *Anthology on Caring.* New York, NY: National League for Nursing Press.

Chinn, P.L. & Kramer, M.K. (1999). *Theory and Nursing: Integrated Knowledge Development* (5th ed.). St Louis, MO: Mosby.

Churchill, S.D. (2007). *Stories of Experience and the Experience of Stories: Methodological Considerations for Qualitative Research in the Wake of Postmodernism.* Paper presented at the 26th Annual International Human Science Research Conference, University of Trento, Rovereto, 13–16 June 2007.

Churchill, S.D. & Wertz, F.J. (2001). An introduction to phenomenological research in psychology: Historical, conceptual and methodological foundations. In K.J. Schneider, J.F.T. Bugentall & J.F. Pierson (Eds.), *The Handbook of Humanistic Psychology: Leading Edges in Theory, Research, and Practice* (pp. 247–262). London, UK: Sage.

Claxton, G. (1997). *Hare Brain, Tortoise Mind: Why Intelligence Increases When You Think Less.* London, UK: Fourth Estate.

Commission on Dignity in Care. (2012). *Delivering Dignity: Securing dignity in care for older people in hospitals and care houses: A report for consultation.* Tavis House, Tavis Square, London, UK. Available from: http://www.nhsconfed. org/PRIORITIES/QUALITY/PARTNERSHIP-ON-DIGNITY/Pages/ Draftreportrecommendations.aspx

Cooley, C. (2004). Do nurses respect themselves enough? *International Journal of Palliative Nursing,* 10 (4), 172.

Cornwell, J & Goodrich, J. (2009). Exploring how to ensure compassionate care in hospital to improve patient experience. *Nursing Times,* 105, (15), 14–16.

Cox, J., Fulford, B., & Campbell, B. (2007). *Medicine of the Person: Faith, Science and Values in Healthcare Provision.* London, UK: Jessica Kingsley Publishers.

Curry, N.R. & Fisher, R. (in press). The role of trust in the development of connectivities amongst rural elders in Britain. *Journal of Rural Studies.*

Dahlberg, H. (2008). *On Movement and Life.* Unpublished paper presented at Kinaesthesia and Motion Conference, Tampere, Finland, October 2–4.

Dahlberg, K. & Segesten, K. (2010). *Hälsa och Värdende: I teori och praxis* [Health and Caring in Theory and Practice] Växel: Natur & Kultur.

Dahlberg, K. & Drew, N. (1997). A lifeworld paradigm for nursing research. *Journal of Holistic Nursing,* 15, 303–317.

Dahlberg, K., Dahlberg, H. & Nystrom, M. (2008). *Reflective Lifeworld Research* (2nd ed.). Lund, Sweden: Studentlitteratur.

Darbyshire, P. (1994). Understanding the life of illness: Learning through the art of Frida Kahlo. *Advances in Nursing Science*, 17 (1), 51–59.

Davis, C. & Schafer, J. (1995). *Between the Heartbeats: Poetry and Prose by Nurses.* Iowa, IA: University of Iowa Press.

Del Barrio, M., Lacunza, M.M., Armendariz, A.C., Margell, M.A. & Asiain, M.C. (2004). Liver transplant patients: Their experience in the intensive care unit – A phenomenological study. *Journal of Clinical Nursing*, 13 (8), 967–976.

Department of Health. (2002). *Shifting the Balance of Power*. London, UK: Department of Health.

Department of Health. (2005). *Creating a Patient-led NHS: Delivering the NHS Improvement Plan.* London, UK: Department of Health.

Department of Health. (2007). *Now I Feel Tall: What a Patient-led NHS Feels Like.* London, UK: HMSO.

Department of Health. (2008). *High Quality Care for All* [Next stage review final report]. Retrieved 05/09/2008 from http://www.dh.gov.uk/en/Publicationsand statistics/Publications/PublicationsPolicyAndGuidance/DH_085825

Department of Health. (2010). *The Essence of Care*. Norwich, UK: The Stationary Office.

Drew, N. & Dahlberg, K. (1995). Challenging a reductionist paradigm for nursing. *Journal of Holistic Nursing*, 13, 332–345

Ekebergh, M. (2007). Lifeworld-based reflection and learning: A contribution to the reflective practice in nursing and nursing education. *Reflective Practice*, 8 (3), 331–343.

Ekebergh, M., Lepp, M. & Dahlberg, K. (2004). Reflective learning with drama in nursing education: A Swedish attempt to overcome the theory praxis gap. *Nurse Education Today*, 24, 622 -628.

Ellis-Hill, C.S., Payne, S. & Ward, C. (2000). Self -body split: Issues of identity in physical recovery following a stroke. *Disability and Rehabilitation*, 22 (16), 725–733.

Entwistle, V., Renfrew, M., Yearly, S., Forrester, J. & Lamont, T. (1998). Lay perspectives: Advantages for health research. *British Medical Journal*, 316 (7129), 463–466.

Epstein, S. (1994). Integration of the cognitive and the psychodynamic unconscious. *American Psychologist*, 49 (8), 709–724.

Eriksson, K. (2006). *The Suffering Human Being*. Chicago, IL: Nordic Studies Press. [English translation of *Den Lidande Manniskan*, Stockholm, Sweden: Liber Forlag, 1994.]

Eriksson, K. (2007). The theory of caritative caring: A vision. *Nursing Science Quarterly*, 20 (3), 201–202.

Evans, M., Ahlzen, R., Heath, I., & Mcnaughton, J. (2008). *Medical Humanities Companion: Volume 1: Symptom*. Oxford, UK: Radcliffe Publishing.

Farran, C.J., Herth, K.A. & Popovich, J.M. (1995). *Hope and Hopelessness: Critical Clinical Constructs*. Thousand Oaks, CA: Sage.

Faulkner, A. & Thomas, P. (2002). User-led research and evidence based medicine. *British Journal of Psychiatry*, 180, 1–3.

Finfgeld, D.L. (2003). Metasynthesis: The state of the art-so far. *Qualitative Health Research*, 13 (7), 893–904.

Finlay, L. (2002). Outing the researcher: The provenance, process and practice of reflexivity. *Qualitative Health Research*, 12 (4), 531–545.

Finlay, L. (2008). A dance between reduction and reflexivity: Explicating the 'phenomenological psychological attitude'. *Journal of Phenomenological Psychology*, 39, 1–32.

Finlay, L. & Gough, B. (Eds.). (2003). *Reflexivity: A Practical Guide for Researchers in Health and Social Science*. Oxford, UK: Blackwell Publishing.

Foucault, M. (1973). *The Birth of the Clinic: Archaeology of Medical Perception* (A.M. Sheridan, Trans.). London and New York: Routledge.

Frank, A. (1995). *The Wounded Storyteller: Body, Illness and Ethics*. Chicago, IL: The University of Chicago Press.

Frank, A.W. (2004). *The Renewal of Generosity: Illness, Medicine and How to Live*. Chicago, IL: University of Chicago Press.

Friedman, N. (2000). *Focusing: Selected Essays 1974-1999*. Bloomington, IN: Xlibris Corporation.

Gadamer, H.G. (1975/1997). *Truth and Method* (2nd rev. ed.). New York, NY: Continuum.

Gadamer, H. (1986). *The Relevance of the Beautiful and Other Essays* (N. Walker, Trans., & R. Bernasconi, Ed.). Cambridge, UK: Cambridge University Press.

Gadamer, H.-G. (1996). *The Enigma of Health* (J. Gaiger & N. Walker, Trans.). Cambridge, UK: Polity Press.

Galvin, K.T., Todres, L. & Richardson, M. (2005). The intimate mediator: A carer's experience of Alzheimer's. *Scandinavian Journal of Caring Sciences*, 19, 2–11.

Gendlin, E.T. (1962). *Experiencing and the Creation of Meaning*. Glencoe, IL: Free Press.

Gendlin, E.T. (1973). Experiential phenomenology. In M. Natanson (Ed.), *Phenomenology and the Social Sciences* (Vol. 1, pp. 281–319). Evanston, IL: Northwestern University Press.

Gendlin, E.T. (1974). The role of knowledge in practice. In G.F. Farwell, N.R. Gamsky & F.M. Mathieu-Coughlan (Eds.), *The counselor's handbook* (pp. 269–294). New York, NY: Intext. Available at http://www.focusing.org/gendlin/docs/gol-2030.html

Gendlin, E.T. (1978). Befindlichkeit: Heidegger and the philosophy of psychology. *Review of Existential Psychology and Psychiatry*, 16, 43–71.

Gendlin, E.T. (1981). *Focusing*. New York, NY: Bantam.

Gendlin, E.T. (1991). Thinking beyond patterns: Body, language and situations. In B. den Outen & M. Moen (Eds.), *The Presence of Feeling in Thought* (pp. 22–151). New York, NY: Peter Lang.

Gendlin, E.T. (1992). The primacy of the body, not the primacy of perception: How the body knows the situation and philosophy. *Man and World*, 25 (3–4), 341–353. Available from: http://www.focusing.org/pdf/primacy_excerpt.pdf [Accessed 15/10/06].

Gendlin, E.T. (1996). *Focusing-Oriented Psychotherapy: A Manual of the Experiential Method*. London, UK: The Guilford Press.

Gendlin, E.T. (1997a). How philosophy cannot appeal to reason and how it can. In D.M. Levin (Ed.), *Language beyond Postmodernism: Saying and Thinking in Gendlin's Philosophy* (pp. 3–41). Evanston, IL: Northwestern University Press.

Gendlin, E.T. (1997b). The Responsive Order: A new empiricism. *Man and World*, 30, 383–411.

Gendlin, E.T. (2004a). Introduction to 'Thinking at the edge'. *The Folio*, 19 (1), 1–10. [Retrieved 15/10/2006 from www.focusing.org/tae-intro.html.]

Gendlin, E.T. (2004b). The new phenomenology of carrying forward. *Continental Philosophy Review*, 37, 127–151.

Giorgi, A. (1997). The theory, practice and evaluation of the phenomenological method as a qualitative research procedure. *Journal of Phenomenological Psychology*, 28 (2), 235–260.

Giorgi, A. (2009). *The Descriptive Phenomenological Method in Psychology: A Modified Husserlian approach*. Pittsburgh, PA: Duquesne University Press.

Giorgi, A. & Giorgi, B. (2003a). Phenomenology. In J.A. Smith (Ed.), *Qualitative Psychology: A Practical Guide to Research Methods* (pp. 25–50). London, UK: Sage.

Giorgi, A. & Giorgi, B. (2003b). The descriptive phenomenological psychological method. In P.M. Camic, J.E. Rhodes & L. Yardley (Eds.), *Qualitative Research in Psychology: Expanding Perspectives in Methodology & Design* (pp. 243–273). Washington, DC: American Psychological Association.

Goffman, E. (1968). *Asylums*. London, UK: Penguin.

Gray, R.E. (2003). Performing on and off the stage: The place(s) of performance in arts-based approaches to qualitative inquiry. *Qualitative Inquiry*, 9 (2), 254–267.

Habermas, J. (1990). *The Philosophical Discourse of Modernity* (F. Lawrence, Trans.). Cambridge, MA: MIT Press.

Halling, S. (2002). Making phenomenology accessible to a wider audience. *Journal of Phenomenological Psychology*, 33 (1), 19–39.

Halling, S., Kunz, G. & Rowe, J. (1994). The contributions of dialogical psychology to phenomenological research. *Journal of Humanistic Psychology*, 34 (1), 109–131.

Harrison, E. (2006). Teaching compassion: Multiple sclerosis and the poetry of Molly Holden. *Nurse Educator*, 31 (3), 103–106.

Heaney, S. (1995). *Opened Ground*. London, UK: Faber.

Heidegger, M . (1927/1962). *Being and Time* (J. Macquarrie & E. Robinson, Trans.). Oxford, UK: Blackwell.

Heidegger, M. (1959/1966). *Gelassenheit* [Discourse on Thinking] (J.M. Anderson & E.H. Freund, Trans.). New York, NY: Harper & Row.

Heidegger, M. (1966). Conversations on a country path. In *Discourse on Thinking* (J.M. Anderson & E.H. Freund, Trans.). New York, NY: Harper & Row.

Heidegger, M. (1969/1973). Kunst und Raum [Art and Space] (C.H. Seibert, Trans.). *Man and World* , 6 (1), 3–5.

Heidegger, M. (1971). *Poetry Language and Thought* (Albert Hofstadter, Trans.). New York, NY: Harper & Row.

Heidegger, M. (1977). *The Question Concerning Technology and Other Essays* (W. Lovitt, Trans.). New York, NY: Harper & Row.

Heidegger, M. (1993a). Building, dwelling, thinking. In D.F. Krell (Ed.), *Basic Writings: Martin Heidegger* (pp. 343–364). London, UK: Routledge.

Heidegger, M. (1993b). Origin of the work of art. In D.F. Krell (Ed.), *Basic Writings: Martin Heidegger*. London, UK: Routledge.

Heidegger, M. (2001). *Zollikon Seminars* (M. Boss, Ed., F. Mayr & R. Askay, Trans.). Evanston, IL: Northwestern University Press.

Hemingway, A. (2011). Lifeworld-led care: Is it relevant for well-being and the fifth wave of public health action? *International Journal of Qualitative Studies on Health and Well-being*, 6. doi: 10.3402/qhw.v6i4.10364.

Hennessey, C., Curry, N., Means, R., Parkhurst, C., Jones, K., Milbourne, P., Jones, R., et al. (2012). *Grey and Pleasant Land? An Interdisciplinary Exploration of*

Peoples' Connectivity in Rural Civic Society. [New Dynamics of Ageing: A UK cross-council Research Programme]. http://ehealth.chiirup.org.uk/greyandpleasant land/ URL Accessed 20th February 2012.

Heron, J. (1996). *Cooperative Inquiry: Research into the Human Condition*. London, UK: Sage.

Hillman, J. (2006). *City and Soul* (Uniform Edition 2). Putnam, CT: Spring Publications.

Hirschfield, J. (1998). *Nine Gates: Entering the Mind of Poetry*. New York, NY: Harper Collins.

Hixon, L. (1989). *Coming Home: The Experience of Enlightenment in Sacred Traditions*. Los Angeles, CA: Tarcher/Perigee.

Hjelmblink, F., Bernsten, C.B., Uvhagen, H., Kunkel, S. & Holstrom, I. (2007). Understanding the meaning of rehabilitation to an aphasic patient through phenomenological analysis: A case study. *International Journal of Qualitative Studies on Health and Well-being*, 2, 93–100.

Holloway I., Sofaer B. & Walker J. (2007). The stigmatisation of people with chronic back pain. *Disability and Rehabilitation*, 29 (18), 1456–1464.

Hossack, A. (1999). The professional, the paraprofessional and the perpetrator. *Journal of Sexual Aggression*, 4 (1), 15–21.

Hunter, L.P. (2002). Poetry as an aesthetic expression for nursing: a review. *Journal of Advanced Nursing* 40 (2), 141–148.

Husserl, E. (1936/1970). *The Crisis of European Sciences and Transcendental Phenomenology. An Introduction to Phenomenological Philosophy* (D. Carr, Trans.). Evanston, IL: Northwestern University Press.

Inwood, M. (1999). *A Heidegger Dictionary*. Oxford, UK: Blackwell.

Jager, B. (2001). The birth of poetry and the creation of a human world. *Journal of Phenomenological Psychology*, 32 (2), 131–152.

Johansson, A. (2008). *Mitt hjärta, mitt liv: Kvinnors osäkra resa mot hälsa efter en hjärtinfarkt* [My heart my life: Women's insecure travel to health after cardial infarction]. Växjö, Sweden: Växjö University, School of Health Sciences and Social Work.

Johansson, A. & Ekebergh, M. (2006). The meaning of well-being and participation in the process of health and care: Women's experiences following a myocardial infarction. *International Journal of Qualitative Studies on Health and Well-being*, 1 (2), 100–108.

Johansson, A., Ekebergh, M. & Dahlberg, K. (2003). Living with experiences following a myocardial infarction. *European Journal of Cardiovascular Nursing*, 2 (3), 229–236.

Jones, K. (2004). The turn to a narrative knowing of persons: Minimalist passive interviewing technique and team analysis of narrative qualitative data. In F. Rapport (Ed.), *New Qualitative Methodologies in Health and Social Care Research* (pp. 35–54). London, UK: Routledge.

Jones, K. (2004). Mission drift in qualitative research or moving toward a systematic review of qualitative studies, moving back to a more systematic review. *The Qualitative Report*, 9 (1), 95–112. Retrieved April 20, 2005, from http://www.nova.edu/ssss/QR/QR9–1/jones.pdf.

Jung, C.G. (1961/1995). *Memories, Dreams, Reflections* (A. Jaffe, Ed.). London, UK: Fontana Press.

Källerwald, S. (2008). *I skuggan av en hotad existens-om den onödiga striden mellan biologi och existens I va°rden av patienter med malignt lymfom* [In the shadow of threatened existence: On the unnecessary battle between biology and existence in the care of malignant lymphoma patients]. Växjö, Sweden: Växjö University Press.

Kegan, R. (1994). *In Over Our Heads: The Mental Demands of Modern Life*. London, UK: Harvard University Press.

Kleinman, A., Das, V. & Lock, M.M. (Eds.). (1997). *Social Suffering*. Berkeley, CA: University of California Press.

Kohlberg, L. (1981). *Essays on Moral Development* (Vol. 1). San Francisco, CA: Harper.

Komesaroff, P. (2001). The many faces of the clinic: A Levinasian view. In S.K. Toombs (Ed.), *Handbook of Phenomenology and Medicine* (pp. 317–330). Dordrecht, The Netherlands: Kluwer Academic Publishers.

Kontos, P.C. & Naglie, G. (2007). Bridging theory and practice: Imagination, the body and person-centred dementia care. *Dementia*, 6 (4), 549–569.

Korzybski, A. (1995). *Science and Sanity: An Introduction to Non-Aristotelian Systems and General Semantics* (5th ed.). Englewood, NJ: Institute of General Semantics.

Krycka, K. (2006). Thinking at the edge: Where theory and practice meet to create fresh understandings. *Indo-Pacific Journal of Phenomenology*, 6, 1–10. [Retrieved 05/07/07 from http://www.ipjp.org/SEmethod/Special_Edition_Method-01_Krycka.pdf]

Kvigne, K. & Kirkevold, M. (2003). Living with bodily strangeness: Women's experiences of their changing and unpredictable body following a stroke. *Qualitative Health Research*, 13 (9), 1291–1310.

Laing, R.D. (1960/2010). *The Divided Self: An Existential Study in Sanity and Madness* (3rd ed.). London, UK: Penguin Classics.

Lakoff, G. & Johnson, M. (1999). *Philosophy in the Flesh: The Embodied Mind and its Challenge to Western Thought*. New York, NY: Basic Books.

Levinas, E. (1974/1981). *Otherwise than Being, or, Beyond Essence* (A. Lingis, Trans.). The Hague, The Netherlands: Martinus Nijhoff.

Levinas, E. (1969/1987). *Totality and Infinity* (A. Lingis, Trans.). Pittsburgh, PA: Duquesne University Press.

Logstrup, K.E. (1995). *Metaphysics II* (R.L. Dees, Trans.). Milwaukee, WI: Marquette University.

Logstrup, K.E. (1997). *The Ethical Demand*. Notre Dame, IN: University of Notre Dame Press.

Lundgren, I. & Dahlberg, K. (2002). Midwives' experience of the encounter with birthing women. *International Journal of Midwifery*, 18, 155–164.

MacDonald, J.B. (1981). Theory, practice and the hermeneutic circle. *Journal of Curriculum Theorizing*, 3 (2), 130–138.

Madden, P. (1990). Rhymes and reasons. *Nursing Times*, 86, 64–65.

Martinsen, K. (2006). *Care and Vulnerability*. Oslo, Norway: Akribe.

Marx, K. (1977). *Capital* (3 vols.). New York, NY: Random House.

Medved, M.I. & Brockmier, J. (2008). Continuity amid chaos: Neurotrauma, loss of memory, and sense of self. *Qualitative Health Research*, 18 (4), 469–479.

Melia, K. (1987). *Learning and Working: The Occupational Socialisation of Nurses*. London, UK: Tavistock.

Merleau-Ponty, M. (1964). *The Primacy of Perception* (J. Edie, Ed.). Evanston, IL: Northwestern University Press.

Merleau-Ponty, M. (1945/1962). *Phenomenology of Perception* (C. Smith, Trans.), London, UK: Routledge

Merleau-Ponty, M. (1964/1968). *The Visible and the Invisible* (A. Lingis, Trans.). Evanston, IL: Northwestern University Press.

Merleau-Ponty, M. (1960/1987). *Signs* (R. McCleary, Trans.). Evanston, IL: Northwestern University Press.

Metz, D.H. (2000). Mobility of older people and their quality of life. *Transport Policy*, 7, 149–152.

Mienczakowski, J., Smith, L. & Morgan, S. (2002). Seeing words, hearing feelings: Ethnodrama and the performance of data. In D. Bagley & M.B. Cancienne (Eds.), *Dancing the Data*. New York, NY: Peter Lang.

Moran, D. (2000). *Introduction to Phenomenology* London, UK: Routledge.

Morse, J.M. (2000). On comfort and comforting. *American Journal of Nursing*, 100 (9), 34–38.

Morse, J.M. (2007). *Why humanized health care? Plenary address* [Saiyud Niymviphat Lecture] Proceedings of the First Asian International Conference on Humanized Health Care, Khon Kaen, Thailand Dec 3–5 2007, pp. 74–81.

Morse, J.M. (2012). *Qualitative Health Research: Creating a New Discipline*. Wallnut Creek, CA: Left Coast Press.

Morse, J.M. & Johnson, J.L. (1991). *The Illness Experience: Dimensions of Suffering*. London, UK: Sage.

Moustakas, C. (1994). *Phenomenological Research Methods*. London, UK: Sage.

Mugerauer, R. (2008). *Heidegger and Homecoming: The Leitmotif in the Later Writings*. Toronto, Canada: University of Toronto Press.

Murray, C.D. & Harrison, B. (2004). The meaning and experience of being a stroke survivor: An interpretative phenomenological analysis. *Disability and Rehabilitation*, 26 (13), 808–816.

Murray, E.L. (1986). *Imaginative Thinking and Human Existence*. Pittsburgh, PA: Duquesne University Press.

Newman, M.A. (1994). *Health as Expanding Consciousness* (2nd ed.). New York, NY: National League for Nursing.

Newman, M.A. (1999). The rhythm of relating in a paradigm of wholeness. *Image: The Journal of Nursing Scholarship*, 31 (3), 227–230.

NHS Executive. (1999). *Patient and Public Involvement in the New NHS*. Leeds, UK: Department of Health.

Nordenfelt, L. (1995). *On the nature of health: An action theoretic approach*. Dordrecht, The Netherlands: Reidel.

Nordgren, L., Asp, M. & Fagerberg, I. (2007). Support as experienced by men living with heart failure in middle age: A phenomenological study. *International Journal of Nursing Studies*, 45 (9), 1344–1354.

Nortvedt, P. (1996). *Sensitive Judgement Nursing, Moral Philosophy and the Ethics of Care*. Oslo, Norway: Tano Aschehoug.

Nortvedt, P. (2001). Needs, closeness and responsibilities: An inquiry into some rival moral considerations in nursing care. *Nursing Philosophy*, 2, 112–121.

Nussbaum, M. (1990). *Loves Knowledge: Essays on the Philosophy and Literature*. Oxford, UK: Oxford University Press.

Nussbaum, M.C. & Sen, A.K. (1993). *The Quality of Life* (1st ed.). Oxford, UK: Oxford University Press.

Nyström, M., Dahlberg, K. & Carlsson, G. (2003). Non-caring encounters at an emergency unit: A lifeworld hermeneutic analysis of an efficiency-driven organization. *International Journal of Nursing Studies*, 40, 761–769.

Office Department of Health. (2005). *Creating a Patient-led NHS, Delivering the NHS Improvement Plan*. London, UK: Department of Health.

Öhlen, J. (2003). Evocation of meaning through poetic condensation of narratives in empirical phenomenological inquiry into human suffering. *Qualitative Health Research*, 13 (4), 557–566.

Oliver, M. (2004). *Wild Geese: Selected Poems*. [Bloodaxe World Poets Series 2]. Tarset, UK: Bloodaxe.

Parkhurst, G., Galvin, K., Musselwhite, C., Phillips, J., Shergold, I. & Todres, L. (2012). *A Continuum for Understanding the Mobility of Older People* [Working Paper]. Bristol, UK: University of the West of England. Available from http://eprints.uwe.ac.uk/16952/

Parliamentary and Health Service Ombudsman. (2011). *Care and Compassion? Report of the Health Service Ombudsman on Ten Investigations into NHS Care of Older People*. London, UK: The Stationery Office. Available from http://www.official-documents.gov.uk

Parse, R. (1981). *Man-Living-Health: A Theory of Nursing*. New York, NY: John Wiley and Sons.

Parsons, T. (1951). *The Social System*. London, UK: Routledge and Kegan Paul.

Pask, E.J. (2005). Self sacrifice, self transcendence and nurses' professional self. *Nursing Philosophy*, 6, 247–254.

Phinney, A. (2002). Fluctuating awareness and breakdown of the illness narrative in dementia. *Dementia*, 1 (3), 329–344.

Polanyi, M. (1996). *The Tacit Dimension*. Garden City, NY: Doubleday.

Polkinghorne, D. (2004). *Practice and the Human Sciences: The Case for a Judgement Based Practice of Care*. Albany, NY: SUNY.

Raingruber, B. (2009). Assigning poetry reading as a way of introducing students to qualitative data analysis. *Journal of Advanced Nursing*, 65 (8), 1753–1761.

Reason, P. (Ed.). (1994). *Participation in Human Inquiry*. London, UK; Sage.

Reed-Danahay, D. (2001). 'This is your home now': Conceptualising location and dislocation in a dementia unit. *Qualitative Research*, 1 (1), 47–63.

Riley, J.M., Beal, J., Levi, O. & McCausland, M.P. (2002). Revisioning nursing scholarship. *Journal of Nursing Scholarship*, 34 (4), 383–389.

Rogers, M.E. (1980). Nursing: A science of unitary man. In J. Riehl and C. Roy (Eds.), *Conceptual Models for Nursing Practice* (2nd ed., pp. 329–337). Norwalk, CT: Appleton Century Crofts.

Rolfe, G. (1998). *Expanding Nursing knowledge. Understanding and Researching Your Own Practice*. Oxford, UK: Butterworth Heinemann.

Rolfe, G., Freshwater, D. & Jasper, M. (2001). *Critical Reflection for Nursing and the Helping Professions: A User's Guide*. Basingstoke, UK: Palgrave.

Romanyshyn, R.D. (1989). *Technology as Symptom and Dream*. London, UK: Routledge.

Rosenhan, D.L. (1973). On being sane in insane places. *Science*, 17 (70), 250–258.

Safranski, R. (1999). *Martin Heidegger: Between Good and Evil* (E. Osers, Trans.). Cambridge, MA: Harvard University Press.

Sandelowski, M. (1998). Writing a good read: Strategies for re-presenting qualitative data. *Research in Nursing & Health*, 21 (4), 375–382.

Schon, D. (1983). *The Reflective Practitioner*. New York, NY: Basic Books.

Schuster, S. (1994). Haiku poetry and student nurses: An expression of feelings and perceptions. *Journal of Nursing Education*, 33, 95–96.

Schütz, A. (1944). The stranger: An essay in social psychology. *American Journal of Sociology*, 49 (6), 499–507.

Sells, D., Topor, A., & Davidson, L. (2004). Generating coherence out of chaos: examples of the utility of empathic bridges in phenomenological research. *Journal of Phenomenological Research*, 35 (2), 253–271.

Sheets-Johnstone, M. (1999). *The primacy of movement*. Amsterdam/ Philadelphia: John Benjamins.

Shengold, L. (1998). *Soul Murder: The Effects of Childhood Abuse and Deprivation*. London, UK: Karnac Books.

Shergold, I., Parkhurst, G. & Musselwhite, C. (2012). Rural car dependence: An emerging barrier to community activity for older people? *Transport Planning and Technology*, 35 (1), 69–85.

Sinason, V. (2011). *Trauma, Dissociation and Multiplicity: Working on Identity and Selves*. London, UK: Routledge.

Smith, S.J. & Lloyd, R.J. (2006). Promoting vitality in health and physical education. *Qualitative Health Research*, 16 (2), 245–267.

Social Care Institute for Excellence. (2008). *Putting People First*. [Retrieved 21 January 2011 from http://www.scie.org.uk/partnerscouncil/meetings/feb08/concordat.pdf]

Spence, D. (1982). *Narrative Truth and Historical Truth*. New York, NY: Norton.

Spiegelberg, E. (1981). *The Phenomenological Movement: A Historical Introduction. (Phaenomenologica)*. (2nd ed.). Dordrecht, The Netherlands: Kluwer Academic.

Spry, T. (2001). Performing autoethnography: An embodied methodological praxis. *Qualitative Inquiry*, 7 (6), 706–732.

Stockwell, F. (1984). *The Unpopular Patient*. Beckenham, UK: Croom Helm.

Stowe, A. (1996). Learning from literature: Novels, plays, short stories, and poems in nurse education. *Nurse Educator*, 21, 16–19.

Svanström, R. (2008). *The everyday life of dementia*. Unpublished manuscript.

Svenaeus, F. (2000). *The Hermeneutics of Medicine and the Phenomenology of Health: Steps Towards a Philosophy of Medical Practice*. London, UK: Kluwer Academic Publishers.

Taylor, C. (1985). *Philosophy and the Human Sciences – Philosophical Papers 2*. Cambridge, UK: Cambridge University Press.

The Patients Association. (2009). *Patients . . . not numbers, People . . . not statistics*. Harrow, UK: The Patients Association.

Todres, L. (1998). The qualitative description of human experience: The aesthetic dimension. *Qualitative Health Research*, 8 (1), 121–127.

Todres, L. (1999). The bodily complexity of truth-telling in qualitative research: Some implication of Gendlin's philosophy. *Humanistic Psychologist*, 23 (3), 283–300.

Todres, L. (2000a). Embracing ambiguity: Transpersonal development and the phenomenological tradition. *Religion and Health*, 39 (3), 227–237.

Todres, L. (2000b). Writing phenomenological-psychological descriptions: An illustration attempting to balance texture and structure. *Auto/Biography*, 3 (1 and 2), 41–48.

Todres, L. (2003). Humanising forces: Phenomenology in science; psychotherapy in technological culture. *Counselling and Psychotherapy Research*, 3 (3), 196–203.

Todres, L. (2004). The meaning of understanding and the open body: Some implications for qualitative research. *Existential Analysis*, 15 (1), 38–55.

Todres, L. (2005). Clarifying the life-world: Descriptive phenomenology. In I. Holloway (Ed.), *Qualitative Research in Health Care*. Maidenhead, UK: Open University Press.

Todres, L. (2007). *Embodied Enquiry: Phenomenological Touchstones for Research Psychotherapy and Spirituality*. Basingstoke, UK: Palgrave Macmillan.

Todres, L. (2008). Being with that: The relevance of embodied understanding for practice. *Qualitative Health Research*, 18 (11), 1566–1573.

Todres, L., Fulbrook, P. & Albarran, J. (2000). On the receiving end: A hermeneutic phenomenological analysis of a patient's struggle to cope while going through intensive care. *Nursing in Critical Care*, 5 (6), 277–287.

Todres, L. & Galvin, K. (2005). Pursuing both breadth and depth in qualitative research: Illustrated by a study of the experience of intimate caring for a loved one with Alzheimer's disease. *International Journal of Qualitative Methods*, 4 (2), Article 2. Retrieved November 24, 2005, from http://www.ualberta.ca/~ijqm/backissues/4–2//pdf/todres.pdf.

Todres, L. & Holloway, I. (2004). Descriptive phenomenology: Life-world as evidence. In F. Rapport (Ed.), *New Qualitative Methodologies in Health and Social Care Research* (pp. 79–98). London, UK: Routledge.

Toombs, K. (1993). *The Meaning of Illness: A Phenomenological Account of the Different Perspectives of Physician and Patient* [Philosophy and Medicine, 42]. Boston, MA: Kluwer Academic Publishers.

Toombs, S.K. (Ed.). (2002). *Handbook of Phenomenology and Medicine* (Vol. 68) [Philosophy and Medicine Series]. London, UK: Springer.

Triestman, J. (1986). Teaching nursing care through poetry. *Nursing Outlook*, 34, 83–87.

Trivedi, P. & Wykes, T. (2002). From passive subjects to equal partners: Qualitative review of user involvement in research. *British Journal of Psychiatry*, 181, 468–472.

Turner, S. (1994). *The Social Theory of Practices*. Chicago, IL: University of Chicago Press.

Van den Berg, J. (1955). *The Phenomenological Approach to Psychiatry*. Springfield, IL: Charles C. Thomas.

Van den Berg, J.H. (1972a). *Psychology of the Sickbed*. Pittsburgh, PA: Duquesne University Press.

Van den Berg, J.H. (1972b). *A Different Existence*. Pittsburgh, PA: Duquesne University Press.

Van Manen, M. (1994). *Researching Lived Experience: Human Science for an Action-Sensitive Pedagogy*. London, Canada: Althouse Press.

Van Manen, M. (1999a). The pathic nature of inquiry and nursing. In I. Madjar & J. Walton (Eds.), *Nursing and the Experience of Illness: Phenomenology in Practice* (pp. 17–35). London, UK: Routledge.

Van Manen, M. (1999b). *The Practice of Practice*. Retrieved 11/02/2010 from www.phenomenologyonline.com/max/articles/practice.html.

Van Manen, M. (2006). Writing qualitatively, or the demands of writing. *Qualitative Health Research*, 16 (5), 713–722.

Watson, J. (1996). Watson's theory of transpersonal caring. In P. Walker & B. Neuman (Eds.), *Blueprint for Use of Nursing Models: Education, Research,*

Practice and Administration (pp. 141–184). New York, NY: National League for Nursing.

Watson, J. (2011). *Human Caring Science: A Theory of Nursing* (2nd ed.). London, UK: Jones & Bartlett

Weber, M. (1963). *The Sociology of Religion*. Boston, MA: Beacon.

Weems, M. (2009). The E in poetry stands for Empathy: Poetic enquiry and phenomenological research-the practice of 'embodied interpretation'. In M. Prendergast, C. Leggo & P. Sameshima (Eds.), *Poetic Inquiry: Vibrant Voices in the Social Sciences* (pp. 133–146). Rotterdam, The Netherlands: Senses Publishers.

Widäng, I., Fridlund, B. & Märtenson, J. (2008). Women patients' perceptions of integrity within health care: A phenomenographic study. *Journal of Advanced Nursing*, 61 (5), 540–548.

Wilber, K. (1995). *Sex, ecology, spirituality: The spirit of evolution*. Boston, MA: Shambhala.

Williams, A.M. & Irurita, V.F. (2004). Therapeutic and non-therapeutic interpersonal interactions: The patient's perspective. *Journal of Clinical Nursing*, 13 (7), 806–815.

Willis, P. (2004). From 'the things themselves' to a 'feeling of understanding': Finding different voices in phenomenological research. *Indo-Pacific Journal of Phenomenology*, 4 (1), 1–13.

Willis, P. (2005). Mythopoetic communities of practice in postgraduate educational research. In T. Stehlik & P. Carden (Eds.), *Beyond Communities of Practice: Theory as Experience* (pp. 47–66). Brisbane, Australia: Post Press.

Young, V. (2000). *Good enough nursing: an exploration of the ways that nurses negotiate interprofessional relationships in managing critical incidents*. Unpublished dissertation, University of Luton. [Cited in Young, V. (2002). Pieces of Time. *Nursing Philosophy*, 3, 90–103.]

Ziebland, S. (2004). The importance of being expert: The quest for cancer information on the internet. *Social Science and Medicine*, 59, 1783–1793.

Index

abiding expanse 65, 69, 71, 75, 80, 82–3
academic 2,131, 181
ache 113
action 132, 53, 132, 135–138, 140–1, 145, 148, 172, 176, 179, 181
addictions 111
adjusting: experience of 6, 47, 52
adventurous horizons 80–2
advocacy 7, 47, 52, 59–63
aesthetic i, ix, 35, 48, 49, 122, 131–3, 137, 147, 150–2, 157–9, 161–2, 164, 167, 168
ageing 67, 125
agency 5, 11–12, 13, 20, 47, 54, 55, 63, 90, 109, 111; human agency 9, 37–38
agenda 2, 5, 21, 178; personal agendas 174, 176
agitation 99; agitated mood 107
alienation 9, 14, 24, 100, 104–5
aliveness 72, 85, 143–4, 151, 158, 162, 163–7, 174
aloneness 14, 59, 71, 73, 174
alterity 174
Alzheimer's disease 6, 18, 25, 40, 42–7, 49, 53, 54, 60–2, 133, 167
ambiguity 177; ambiguous 39, 92, 93, 174–5, 177
ambivalence 102; ambivalence scene 174
analysis 30, 48, 49, 71, 79, 119, 136, 165, 167; phenomenological analysis 48, 154; see also phenomenology
analytical 34, 148, 151
anger 51, 63, 106, 173
anguish 25, 92, 102, 177
anomie 9

anthropology: anthropological 128
anxiety 27, 29, 62, 71, 101, 107, 109, 111, 115, 173; annihilatory anxiety 111
application 50, 81, 135, 148, 149, 161–2, 165, 168, 170, 171, 179; instrumental application 170
architecture 17–18
Arendt, H. 12, 184
Aristotle 138, 184
art 91, 136–8, 143, 147; arts ix, 32, 131, 137, 148, 183; artist 144–5
arthritis 109
Ashworth, P. x, 47, 79, 184
assessment 11, 32
astronomy 123
at-homeness 17, 20, 66, 71, 72, 79, 80–2, 87–8,116–7, 125, 127–9
attitude: judgemental 177
attraction: interpersonal 76, 80, 85–7, 10–4
audiences 47, 64, 150, 155, 161, 167–8
authenticity 71; authentic 9, 71–2, 74, 159, 164, 179
autobiography: autobiographical 17
aversion 99, 103–5, 107
awareness 10, 19, 41, 51, 59–60, 110, 112, 157, 175, 178; felt awareness 175

Bachelard, G. 142,184
bedridden 180
Being and Time 71, 73, 79, 84, 189
being: being with 9, 87, 103, 140; being for 140; integration of being and knowing 133 (see integration)
being-in-the-world 18, 65, 75, 143

belonging 14–15, 17, 74–6, 80, 82, 84, 86, 87, 104, 92, 104–5
Benner, P. 135, 148, 157, 179, 180, 182, 185
biography: biographical 17
biomedical 19, 23, 35, 38, 94; descriptions 182; model 18, 23, 149
body: as carnal matter 175; as soulful window 176; body-forth 112; body image 30
body object 9, 113, 175, 178; body subject 9, 175; dominance 175; epistemic
body 151; lived body 28, 143–6, 164–5; unreal body 153
boredom 103
Boss, M. 26, 29–30, 72–3, 79, 104, 182, 185, 189
breathing 40, 84, 100, 112, 173
Buber, M. 49, 159, 185

cancer 14, 15, 24, 108, 125
capability: negative capability 142, 143
capacity i, ix, 2–3, 28, 40, 58, 66, 76, 93, 98; developing capacity to care 131–133, 158, 169–70, 183; ethical 148, unspecialised 141
capital: community capital 117
care: capacity i, ix, 66, 98,131, 133, 158, 169–70, 183; directions for 66, 182–3; humanly sensitive care i, 2–3, 37, 46, 66, 98, 114, 133, 135, 147, 149–150, 155–6, 183; human dimensions of care 9, 157; meaning of care 2, 183; non care 2; professional carers 44, 122, 156
Carel, H. 149, 182, 185
caring: practice of 170; caring for well-being 2, 133, 182–3; systems of 5, 9, 20
carry forward 133, 158, 164, 167
Cartesian 164
causality 18, 103
chemotherapy 173
Churchill, S. 30, 167, 186
citizen empowerment 35
citizenship 6, 24, 35, 37, 44
city 129
claustrophobic 99–100, 125
clearing 71, 84, 141; clearing in the forest 140
clinical: encounters 172; gaze 65
coherence: sense of coherence 140–41

comfort 32, 71, 77, 80, 84; as wellbeing dimension 94–6, as related to suffering 113
commodification 137; commodified 171
commonality 6, 14, 35, 159, 174
communicative concern 48,132, 150
compartmentalisation 146
conflict 103, 138
connectivity 118, 128; human connectedness 14, 175; seamless 2
constituents 10, 26, 26–7, 30, 33–4, 76, 79
consumerist 6, 37–8
contemplation 132, 135–6,140–6, 171
continuum; humanising dimensions 1–11; mobilities continuum 120; *see also* mobility well-being and suffering 98
conviviality 122
core value 5–6, 24, 33
creativity: of unspecialisation 135–7, 141, 143, 146
critical care 100
culture 1, 14, 15, 17, 39, 127–9; audit culture 171
cure 2, 9, 177

Dahlberg, K. 2, 23, 25, 30, 32, 40–1, 43, 47, 171, 182
data 34, 124
death 39, 108, 173, 174–175
dehumanising 5, 9, 10–11, 13, 17, 18–20, 24, 26
dementia 19, 41, 51, 53, 96
denial 51, 107, 175
de-personalisation 14; depersonalised 110–11
depletion 94, 114
depression 27, 30, 99, 106–8
description: lifeworld 26–7, 29–30, 48, 64; phenomenological 48, 160; rich 7, 152
despair 99, 101, 103, 105–6, 112, 115
deterministic 18, 96, 110, 114
development: human 114; personal 172, 179; professional 3, 149, 151, 172, 181
diagnosis 14, 45, 107, 110; diagnoses 176
dialectical 129
dialysis: renal dialysis 111
dignity 1, 5, 12, 13–14, 17, 21, 37, 47, 55, 63, 136–7,
dimensions: core 9, 35, 38

dingle 126
disability 17, 154–5
discomfort 51–3, 99, 113–4, 145, 180
dis-coordination 112
dis-ease 18, 95, 113
disempowered 111
disgust 29, 104, 173, 175
disjunction 55, 109, 177
dislocation 5, 7, 15, 17
dispossession 106, 111
dissociation 12, 111, 137
diversity 117, 136–7
dizziness 113
dualism 10, 42; dualistic 19
dwelling: embodied 94–5; existential
    65, 72, 74; identity 91–2;
    intersubjective 86–7; mood 88–9,
    107; temporal 84, 102; spatial
    81–2; prompted to 125; choice to
    125
dwelling-mobility; embodied 95; *gegnet*
    74–5; identity 92; intersubjective 87;
    mood 89; temporal 84; spatial 82,
    theory of wellbeing 69

earth: sky, mortals and divinities 70,
    114; environing 128
ecology: ecological 128
economics 35, 117; economic i, 15, 24,
    36–7, 39, 75, 96, 114–5
education: methodologies 157; resource
    156–7
egocentric 140
einraumen 70
elders; rural 117–8, 127–9
embodied relational understanding 3,
    131–2, 147–152, 155, 170
embodiment: as a humanising
    dimension 5, 11, 18
emotion 12; attunement 29; processing
    58
empathy 14, 61, 115, 147, 149; feeling
    capacities 158; understanding 3, 31,
    64, 132–3, 149, 155–7, 168
empirical 30, 66, 118, 128
emptiness 111; deficient 89
ennui 112
enquiry 145; embodied 162, 179
epistemology 136, 14, 158, 161
    actionable 149; embodied 183;
    frameworks, 6,132, 159, 161, 165
eros 72, 85–6, 103–4, 106; therapeutic
    104; sexual 104
esoteric 177

essence: essential structure 120, 125
estrangement 100
ethics: ethics committee 118
ethnographic study 17
etymology 131
evidence: technical 148
excess 143–4, 151, 160, 164, 166,
    180
excitement 77, 80, 88, 106
exhaustion 99, 112–4
exile: spatial 99–100; interprersonal
    104
existentialism: dwelling 65, 72–4;
    existentials 73, 77, 159;
    homelessness 2, 72; mobility 40, 65,
    72–3; theory of well-being 2, 65–6,
    69, 72–5, 97, 98, 114; tradition 34,
    69, 159
experience: everyday 30, 76, 150, 172,
    181; experience-near 118;
    experiential intricacy 144; 'song of
    experience' 90, 172, 178
expert 45, 179; expertise 44–5, 60, 62,
    177

fatigue 112
feeling: met as human 5; felt
    complexity 165; 'felt sense' 49, 65,
    82, 88, 94–5, 109, 112, 114–5, 139,
    144–5, 151, 164, 166, 167, 171,
    179–181
figural 71; figure/ground 80–1
finitude 39, 71, 73, 98, 177
Finlay, L. 149, 187–8
flourishing 104
flow 25, 40, 42, 57, 65, 72, 74–6, 79,
    83, 85, 95, 148, 179; sense of 132
focusing: the practice of 48, 133, 144,
    166, 179
Foucault, M. 24, 180, 188
four-fold 70
fragility: limits 18; nursing
    openheartedness 178
fragmentation 16, 111, 136, 140
framework: conceptual ix, 1, 3, 5,
    9–11, 22,34, 65, 77–8, 182;
    humanising i, 9, 21; value 5, 9–15,
    17, 19, 21
Frank, A. 24, 38, 180, 188
freedom 9, 12, 31, 36, 38–40, 42–3,
    75, 98, 100–1, 125, 114, 161, 174,
    183; freedom-wound 114
future: blocked future 99, 102–3;
    future orientation 80, 83–4

Gadamer, H-G. ix, 72–3, 132, 158, 161–2, 165, 188
Galvin, K.T. 25, 46, 188, 193, 195
gardens 123
Gelassenheit 73–4, 79, 84, 189
Gendlin, E.T. ix, 48, 132, 136, 143–5, 148, 151, 161–6, 179, 188–9
generalisation 35, 176
geography 117
gestalt 15
Giorgi, A. 48–9, 165, 167, 189
gloom 99, 107–8
Grey and Pleasant Land 189
grounded theory 15–16
guidelines 34, 176
guilt 58–9, 106

Habermas, J. 24, 136–7, 189
Halling, S. 32, 150, 184, 189
hand: and world 24; ready to hand 174, 176–7
harmony 70, 107
hate; of self 106, 109
head: 'head, hand and heart' 3, 132–3, 137, 141–2, 145–8, 150, 155, 179; *see also* 'hand and heart' 146; 'head and heart' 162, 167
healing: resource 19
health: health and social care i, ix 1–2, 5, 13, 32, 35, 62, 65, 104, 107, 131, 160; mental health 108, 111
heart: heartfelt 1, 155, 160, 168–9
Heidegger, M. ix, 9, 24, 26, 38–40, 42, 69, 76, 78–9, 84, 132–3, 136, 139–40, 142–4, 158–9, 164, 172, 174, 176, 188–90, 192–3
heritage 39, 66, 86–8, 115, 124, 126, 128; embodied heritage 133, 172–3, 175–6, 178
hermeneutic 158, 163, 168; hermeneutic circle 31, 191; hermeneutics 71
hermeneutics 144, 162–3, 165
Hillman, J. 129, 190
history 16, 115, 126, 128; personal history 77, 87, 127, 180; historical narrative 25
holism 26, 137; holistic 15, 23, 25–6, 29; holistic perspective 23, 25, 34; holistic meanings 29; holistic knowing 147, 151, 164; holistic nursing 171

Holloway, I. 9, 12, 34, 48–9, 150, 190, 195
homecoming: authentic 71–2, emotional 151, 159–60; Heidegger and 65, 69–73, 75, 78–9, 98, 189, 192–3 (also *see* at-homeness)
homelessness: existential 2, 70–5
homogenisation 5, 11, 13
hopelessness 103, 106
hospital 100, 106, 121, 173–4; anthroposophic hospital 18
hospitality 101, 163, 178, 183; hospitable 17, 131, 145
human: to be human i, 1, 5, 9–10, 12–18, 27; human dimensions 1, 9, 18, 157, 165
human bond 151
humanisation: humanisation of care i, ix, 1, 3, 5–6, 9–22, 65, 133, 182–3; humanising force 6, 32–3
humanities ix, 9, 131, 183; health-related humanities 149
humanity 45; common humanity 49, 115, 133, 156, 158
humiliation 104, 175; humiliation scene 173
Husserl, E. ix, 5, 25–6, 34–5, 76, 79, 190

I am. . . 80, 91–3; 'I am an object or thing' 99, 109–10; 'I am fragmented' 99, 110; 'I am unable' 99, 109; 'I can' 77, 81, 90–2
I and Thou 185; *I in the thou* 31, 49
iatrogenically 115
ideal types 10
identity 14, 80; personal identity 24–5, 55, 77, 90–3, 99, 109–11
ill health; chronic 16, 90; absence of illness 2, 6, 18, 39, 44, 69
imagery 156
imagination: empathic imagination 31, 50, 133, 139, 140, 146, 149, 151, 158–169 (*see also* empathy); imaginative thinking 139
immersion 164; immersion in practice 135–6, 148
implicit: philosophy of implicit entry ix, 143–5, 151, 164, 172, 179; and felt experience 181
impotence 111
imprisoned 99, 101, 158
inauthenticity 71–2

incarcerated 106
incompetence 109
incontinence 60, 61; faecal incontinence 173
inhospitable 100
injury 17, 106, 110, 113
innocence 86; 'songs of innocence' 90, 172, 178
insecurity 13, 41, 72, 110
insider 12, 20, 150; insiderness 5, 11, 12, 18, 20
institutions 5, 14, 24, 106; institutional 13–15, 96, 106, 114, 141, 179
integration: scholarly integration 132, 143; integration of being and knowing 133
integration of knowledge 132, 136, 140–1
intelligence: emotional intelligence 168
interaction 12, 14, 19, 30, 44, 80, 99, 161, 173, 174, 177; social interaction 53; dehumanising interaction 19; interactions 5, 9, 20, 29, 30, 37, 56, 196
interdisciplinary 19, 116, 121
internet 122, 140
interpersonal: world 28, 105,159; attraction 76, 80, 85–7, 104; aversion 103–4; connection 86, 104–5
interpretation: interpretive 48–9, 161, 162, 185; embodied interpretation 46, 48–9, 50–1, 55, 57, 59, 62, 132–3, 147–8, 151–2, 155–8, 165–9
intersubjectivity: intersubjective dimension in well-being theory 80, 99
intertwined 26, 66, 78, 80–1, 96–7, 99, 101, 103, 105–8, 110–12, 129, 135, 177; intertwining 42, 70, 95, 108, 114, 175
intervention 55–6, 59, 174, 175; interventions 9, 106, 185; technical intervention 174
interviews 17, 118–9; interview 47, 49, 118–9; narrative 17
intimacy 7, 14, 24–6, 56–7, 59, 84, 87, 94, 135; intimately human 12; interpersonal
intimacy 39, 47
intravenous lines 100
irritation 63, 107, 113

isolation 11, 14, 32; alienated isolation 99, 105; social isolation 15–6
itchiness 113

Jager, B. 178, 190
Jones, K. 32, 189, 190
journey 5, 25, 44–6, 54, 64, 87–8, 102; personal journey 5, 11,16; through homelessness 71
judgement: judgement based care 31, 174, 193
Jung, C. 92, 190

kinship 71, 76, 80, 86–7, 104–5
knowing: experiential 62–3, 157; holistic 147, 151, 164; kinds of 170; participative 115, 139, 149, 165, 168; propositional 2, 63; 'thick pattern' of 148
knowledge: actionable 46, 131–2, 147–8; complex 147–151; contemplative 135; domains of 135–6, 140, 148; empathic 148; knowledge-in-action 135
knowledge-for-action 135; medical 113; propositional 64, 148, 168; specialised 149; technical 3, 45, 156, 171; sociology of 136

labelling: labelled 12–13
Laing, R.D. 110, 191
landscapes: storied 116
language; body 29; 'more than words can say' 29, 144, 151, 160, 164; poetic
language (also see poetry) 156, 161, 168; as summative 151, 157–8, 161, 163
layered continuity 80, 92–3
leisure 116, 122
lethargy 94, 112
letting-be 41–2, 73–4, 77, 88, 98; letting-be-ness 42, 73–4, 77, 88, 98; also *see gelassenheit*
Levinas, E. ix, 133, 145, 172–3, 178, 191
libido: loss of libido 112
life force 88, 93, 112
life projects 30, 40, 94, 112
lifeworld; beginning place 9, 25; colonisation of 24, 127; constituents 33–4, 76, 79
lifeworld-led care ix, 2, 5–6, 22–3, 30–8, 43–6, 69; lived world 164

lighting: artificial lighting 100
limbo 101, 103
liminal: space 83, 108, 128; mood 108
lived experience 26, 29, 46, 160
locale: rich textured locale 67, 125–6,
    128–9
Logstrup, K.E. 179, 191
loneliness 29, 104–5
longing
loss: of meaning 5, 11, 15; of personal
    journey 5, 11, 16

manic 102
marginality 20, 108, 177, 180
Martinsen, K. 182, 191
Marx, K. 24, 191
mastery 109
meaning: bodily alive meanings 162,
    166; of things 15; of mobility
    116–129; meaning units 119;
    transformed meaning units
    119–20
media 9, 21
mediator 60, 62, 160–1; evocative
    mediator 160
medical model 13, 37
medication 61, 106
memory: loss of 6, 17, 40, 47, 50–1,
    112; valuing 63
mentor: elders as 129
Merleau-Ponty, M. ix, 26, 28, 38, 40,
    79, 133, 144, 164, 172–3, 175,
    191–2
metaphor 113, 158, 159; metaphorical
    ix, 70, 77, 81–3, 86–8, 90, 94–5,
    100–1, 105–6, 109, 137
methodology: approach 30, 48, 117;
    innovation 46, 165;
    phenomenological 46
middle: middle of nowhere 126; middle
    of everywhere 126
mirror-like multidimensional fullness
    80, 89
mobility; continuum 120, 193;
    embodied 93, 95; identity 4, 90,
    109; imaginative 122–3, 125;
    intersubjective 85, 87, 104; literal
    113, 121–6; needs 66, 128; mood
    88, 106; potential 103, 123–4;
    spatial 77, 82, 100, 120, 123–4;
    temporal 77, 83–4, 101; virtual
    122–3, 125
modernity 24, 136, 137, 148; disaster
    of 136–7; dignity of 137

mood 12, 26–7, 29–30, 33–5, 38, 73–4,
    76–7, 79–81, 88–90, 99, 106–8,
    111, 149, 182
morality 136–8, 147
Moran, D. 2, 78, 192
Morse, J.M. 10, 47, 182, 192
movement: bodily 73, 93, 112,
    imagined 81; impairment 112;
    literal 94, 118, 122–3; potential
    85; vitality 40, 43
Mugerauer, R. 70–2, 75, 78, 84,
    192
multiple sclerosis 16, 112
music 84, 86, 123
mutual complementarity 80, 87
mysterious interpersonal attraction
    76, 80, 85–7
mytho-poetic 142

narrative: essential structure 166–7,
    unifying ix, 3, 133, 183
nature: natural world 116–7, 127–8
nausea 51, 113
Newman, M.A. 32, 170, 192
non-reductionist 19
not-knowing 87, 108, 133, 143, 170,
    175, 177
novelty 16, 75, 84, 87, 89, 143
numbness 102, 108, 111
nursing 135, 148, 150, 156, 170–1;
    theory 135, 170, 182
Nussbaum, M. 2, 139, 192

objectivity: objectification 5, 11–12, 20,
    110–1; objectified gaze 133, 172,
    174, 176; of world: 24–5, 137, 161,
    168
old age: mobility 117–8, 120, 123–9,
    rural elders 117–8, 127–9
ontic 70–1, 76–7, 79, 159
ontology 6, 69–72, 75, 79, 91–2, 110,
    133, 159, 160, 170, relational 143;
    insecurity 110; and correspondence
    theory 50, 163, 168
open-heartedness; nursing 133, 171–3,
    176, 181; open heart 170, 172,176,
    178
open-mindedness 171; definition of
    openness 143; openness to future
    42, 74–5, 85
openness to otherness 33, 43, 51, 85,
    131, 133, 149, 163, 177–8
oppression: of blocked future 103
organisations 5

otherness: infinity of 133, 172–4, 178
outsider 12, 104–5, 155
ownness 9, 75

pain 113: chronic pain 106; emotional 108–9; painful closing down 99, 113
paralysis 112
Parse, R. 170, 182, 193
passivity 5, 11–13, 37, 143,
past: as temporality 16, 27, 41, 74, 77, 85, 102, 122, 128, 139
patience: a mood dimension of dwelling 88
patient: patient-centred 36, 37, 43–5, patient-led care ix, 6, 36
peacefulness 74, 80–9
pedagogy 141, 131
persecution 99, 105–6
personhood 12, 19, 38, 47
pets 123
phenomenology; aesthetic 132–3, 147, 150–1, 158–9, 161, 164, 168; attitude 117; case study 6, 30, 47, 154; descriptive 151, 158, 168; existential 159; experiential ix, 48, 64, 65, 78, 151, 162, 168; interpretive 48, 162; research findings 147, 150–1; tradition ix, 2, 34, 69, 139, 171, 182; as a way of seeing 159
phenomenon: structure of 125, 150,
philosophy: continental 171; of care 6, 36; of entry into the implicit 141, 143–4, 151, 172; see also implicit; of the person 6, 36; lifeworld-oriented 182
phronesis 132, 136, 138–140, 147, 179; see also practical wisdom
place: sense of place 5, 11, 17–18, 67, 82, 128; storied place 126
play: in Gadamer 142, 161
poetry 133, 150–1, 156–61, 163, 168–9
poignancy 46, 156, 173, 176
Polanyi, M. 179, 193
policies 6, 31, 36, 39, 171, 183; documents i, 21, 36, 43–4, 187; political 15, 31, 35–7, 43–4, 60–1, 179–80; political dimensions of well-being 39, 96, 114
Polkinghorne, D. 45–6, 138–9, 148, 156–7, 193
portal 66, 117, 119–25, 128

possessed: by alien forces 111
possibility: of suffering 99–112; of well-being 31, 39, 65, 69–70–7, 79–99; non deterministic 110
postmodernity 136–7, 148
powerlessness 177
practical wisdom 46, 63, 132, 135, 138–9, 140, 179; see also phronesis
practice: caring 6, 30, 114, 131–141, 147–8; see also caring; epistemological 183; development 131; experiential 144, 164; evidence based 147; humanly sensitive 64; nursing 147, 156, 170, 178; see also nursing; responsiveness 133, 172, 176–8; 'readiness to hand'('zuhandensein') 174, 176; reflective 31, 33–4, 149
pre-reflective 26, 29, 94, 141, 178
presence: being 166; palpable 157, 168; physical 177; presencing 47
present; elusive 99, 102–3, 107; present centredness 80, 84
primordial 28, 73, 95, 175, 178
privacy 14, 17, 55, 104, 125
psychiatry 14, 25, 43
psychology: developmental 139; of the sickbed 41
psychotherapy 73, 162

qualitative research 10–21; 25, 32, 46, 132, 147, 150, 156, 162, 164, 169
quidity 150

rationality 138–9, 158, 169, 177; embodied 139
reductionism 9, 18, 37 view of the body 5, 11, 18–19
relationality 26, 178
releasement 98; see also letting-be-ness
reminiscence 123
renewal 80, 84–5, 95
re-presentation 131, 150, 156, 158, 167, 169
Research Councils UK 116
research: collaboration 116; findings 132–3, 147, 150–2, 157, 158; lifeworld-oriented 131, 152; questions 117–8; 'research worker' 142; translational 150
resonance 34, 49, 128, 151; personal 49, 161; evocative 167; validity 47–50, 64, 168

resource: educational 156–7; reflective 45, 157
respite: 'no respite' 99, 102
restlessness 72, 95–103, 107, 113
retirement 56, 125
reverie 142
reversibility 175; *see* also body subject and body object
rhizome 116,139,
rhododendrons 125
Romanyshyn, R.D. 24, 193
roommaking 70, 74; *see* also *einraumen*
roomless 99, 100
rootedness 65, 75–6, 79
routines 17–18, 54
rupture 71, 104–5, 107, 113

sameness 17, 87, 174, 177
scholarship 131–2, 135–42; contemplative 141–6
science: caring science 64; human science 31, 133, 168, 183; natural science 136
'scientific concern' 48, 150; social science 117
seasons 25, 27, 54, 88–9, 123, 127
self: self-betrayal 110; self-belief 90; self-care 7, 54–5; self-cutting 174; self-disgust 173, 175; self-efficacy 91, 109; self-forgetting 110; self-hate 109; self-hood 19, 79
sense of agency 12, 54
sense of dislocation 5, 15
sense of personal journey 5
sense of place 5, 11, 17, 18, 67, 82, 128
sense-making 5, 11, 15, 20, 34
sensitivity: ethical 151
sensitisation 56, 77, 114
shame 104, 153, 155, 173, 175
Sheets-Johnstone, M. 40, 194
shopping 119, 122
sick role 13, 112
signs: and symptoms 18, 66, 114
Skype 122
sleep 95, 100, 108
social: connection 14; engineering 137; inclusion 128
sociology: of knowledge 136; perspectives 9
soul: soul murder 109, 194; soul suicide 109

South West England 118
space: traverse of 118, 121, 124
spatiality 9, 26, 27, 29, 33–4, 38, 73, 76–7, 79, 80, 98–100, 117, 128, 159, 182
specialisation 1–2, 9, 23–4, 65, 127, 135, 137, 141–3, 145–6, 149, 176–6; overspecialisation 17, 135
spectrum: of humanising dimensions 10–12, 19–20; of spatial mobility 123; of
sufferings 114
speech; impaired speech 112
spirituality 18, 38
spontaneity 177
stagnation: temporal 101
statistics i, 1, 12, 15–16, 35, 104, 110
stigmatisation 12, 53
story tellers 15
stranger 14, 17, 104–5, 152
stroke 132, 148, 152–4, 167
structure: general phenomenological 168; essential 120, 125
studies: case 30, 47, 154; empirical 19, 128; phenomenological 6, 30
subjectivity 12, 20, 25–6, 32, 137, 161, 174; well-being 78; body 175
suffering, 2–3, 65–6, 98–115; economic 115; social 115; psychological 115
support groups 15, 23, 32, 63–4, 169
survey 118
Svenaeus, F. 23, 28, 30, 32, 38–9, 45, 71, 182, 194
swallowing: difficulties in 112
Sweden 18, 36
symptoms 16, 18–19, 30, 66, 114, 182
synthesis i, 3, 23, 48, 133
systemic 110

tacit 77, 95, 179
targets 1, 129
teaching 142
techne 138
technology: progress 6, 9, 16, 24, 32–3, 137, 140; spirit of 24, 140; technologies 23, 32, 120, 122
telephone 18, 119, 122
television 123

temporality: as a lifeworld constituent 9, 16, 26–7, 29, 33–4, 38; in relation to well being 41, 73–81, 98; in relation to suffering 99, 159, 182; rhythm 124
terror 105–6
text 49, 155, 160, 165–7
texture: in relation to aesthetic phenomenology 48, 150–1, 158, 162
theory: existential 2, 65–6, 69, 72, 75, 97, 98, 114; grounded 15–16; lifeworld 26, 38; dwelling-mobility 69, 127, nursing 170; of wellbeing 6, 39, 69–77, 97–8, 114, 127, 183
thinking: calculative 142–3; contemplative 132, 142–3; experiential 139; 'thinking at the edge' 144, 162, 188, 191
Todres, L. i, 10, 20, 25, 31–2, 34–5, 39, 42, 46, 48–9, 114, 141, 148, 150, 156, 162, 179, 188, 193–5
togetherness 5, 11, 14, 70, 75, 86
tolerance 106
Toombs, S.K. 23, 38–9, 45, 72–3, 160, 182, 191, 195
touchstones: experiential 10, 147, 179
transcript 119
transpersonal 92
transport 66, 117–22, 124; public 121, trauma 102, 174
tremor 112
trust 58, 94, 105–6, 141, 177, 181
truth: narrative 35; objective truth 15, 35, 148; questions of 137, 142, 148, 159
turning: *Kehre* 73
twilight 114

uncanniness 71; *see also* unhomely
uncovering 140, 178, 181
understanding: background 165; embodied 133, 179, 181; felt 167; 'felt senses' 179; lived 179; logical 160; touched 133
unhomely 18, 30, 106; *unheimleich* 71
uniqueness: in relation to humanising care 5, 11, 13–14
University of Western England 118
unpredictability 113, 138, 177
unspecialisation 135–146
unworthiness: sense of 106, 109–10
user involvement 13

validity 48, 50, 136–7, 168; as application 168; resonant 47, 50, 64, 168; also *see* resonance
value: base 9, 20, 22, 30; core 5–6, 24, 33; absolute 10
vampires 111
Van Den Berg, J.H. 23, 26, 28, 41, 195
Van Manen, M. 46, 48, 135, 141–2, 148, 160, 195
variation: in relation to commonality 6, 35, 76–7, 81, 114, 122, 125, 171; variations of well-being 80: variations of suffering 99
vibrancy: grounded 80, 95–6
vicious circle 110
vignettes 133, 145, 171–81
vitality 18, 36, 40–3, 80, 88, 93–6, 104, 107, 112, 141
vocabulary: descriptive 66, 114; for care 182; for suffering 99,114; for well-being 80, 97
vulnerability: caring 98–115; bodily 116, 180; existential 39, 42–44, 73, 98, 115, 170, 177; shared 175, 181

Wales 118
weakness: muscle weakness 112
webcam 122
well-being: experiential 78, 96, kinds and levels of 65–6, 75–76; 78–97; priorities 66; spatial 116, 128; *see* also dwelling-mobility theory of well-being
Wertz, F. 30, 186
wholeness 70, 156; sense of the whole 48, 145, 165, 183
Wilber, K. 3, 136–7, 196
wildlife 123
Willis, P. 48, 142, 149, 151, 164, 196
withdrawal: in relation to suffering 112
witness: bearing witness 103
world-to-consciousness 25–6
wound: *see* freedom-wound

Zollikon seminars 71, 79, 189
zuhandensein 176–7, 177; *see* also ready to hand

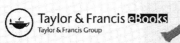